SELF-CARE FOR LONG COVID: A FUNCTIONAL MEDICINE GUIDE

SUSANNA HUHTINIEMI, MSc

This book was published thanks to free support and training from:
TCKPublishing.com

CONTENTS

INTRODUCTION: THE PATH AHEAD

In the ongoing global battle against Long COVID, I've witnessed firsthand the challenges many face in their quest for recovery. With over two decades dedicated to unraveling the intricate mechanisms of illness and health, this book is my attempt to offer a fresh perspective on Long COVID and provide a transformative path towards reclaiming your health. It's a blend of my firm foundation in biochemistry and cell-level processes with the healing abilities of functional medicine informed by nutrition.

While the content is accurate, detailed, and grounded in scientific understanding, it is crafted to be accessible to all, even individuals without a medical background.

Long COVID isn't merely a medical condition; it's a life-altering experience. Many have navigated countless doctor visits, sought answers in medications, and experienced the frustrations of prolonged symptoms without relief. But within these pages lies a different approach, a turning point. Here, self-care becomes a powerful tool for healing, reducing dependence on frequent doctor visits.

It's time to shatter the confines of traditional medical routes. Let's step into a world where self-care, bolstered by functional medicine, becomes our beacon. This is about taking control, initiating healing, and crafting a new narrative for your well-being.

The book is divided into eleven chapters. Chapter 1, "Unveiling Long COVID," delves into the prevalence and mechanisms of Long COVID. Chapter 2, "The Power of Functional Medicine," gives insight about functional medicine's healing philosophy. The subsequent chapters from 3 to 10 are dedicated to providing detailed information and treatment strategies for each of the main symptoms associated with Long COVID. Chapter 11, "Your Comprehensive Care Plan," summarizes and integrates what you have learnt throughout the book into a holistic approach. Finally, in the Appendices, you will find additional resources, including treatment plan charts and meal planning tools.

Together, let's embark on this transformative journey, where healing becomes more than a hope — it becomes your reality.

Welcome to Self-Care for Long Covid: A Functional Medicine Guide.

Chapter 1. Unveiling Long COVID: A Closer Look at the Invisible Battle

Introduction

Long COVID is a term that has emerged from the global struggle with the SARS-CoV-2 virus, which causes the disease known as COVID-19. This condition, also referred to as post-acute sequelae of SARS-CoV-2 infection (PASC), continues to puzzle scientists and clinicians alike, with its broad spectrum of lingering symptoms and the diversity of its potential triggers. Before we delve into the potential causes of Long COVID, let's first understand the basics of how the SARS-CoV-2 virus interacts with the body.

How SARS-CoV-2 Infects the Body

The virus primarily targets cells lining the respiratory tract, from the nose and sinuses to the lungs. Using its signature spike protein, the virus latches onto angiotensin-converting enzyme 2 (ACE2) receptors on the surface of these respiratory epithelial cells.

ACE2 Receptors

Under normal conditions, the ACE2 receptor plays a key role in blood pressure regulation and cardiovascular homeostasis. It converts the hormone angiotensin II into angiotensin 1-7, which lowers blood pressure by promoting vasodilation. This counters some effects of the renin-angiotensin system that lead to vasoconstriction and fluid retention, thus helping maintain balance. SARS-CoV-2 exploits ACE2 to gain entry into cells, disrupting its normal function. ACE2 is found in cells throughout the body, but is particularly abundant in the cells of the respiratory and cardiovascular systems. Once the spike protein binds to ACE2, the virus fuses with the host cell membrane and enters the cell. From there, it hijacks the cell's machinery to replicate itself, ultimately leading to cell death and damage in the airways and lungs.

The initial site of infection, such as the nasal passages versus deep lung tissue, may determine the subset of symptoms that manifest. For example, people with more upper respiratory infection may experience more loss of taste and smell. Those with deeper lung involvement can develop pneumonia.

INDIVIDUAL VULNERABILITIES

Certain individuals may be more vulnerable to SARS-CoV-2 infection due to increased expression of ACE2 receptors. Elderly males tend to have higher ACE2 levels, likely due to age-related hormonal changes, comorbidities, and medication use. Patients taking ACE inhibitor and ARB medications (angiotensin receptor blockers) used to treat cardiovascular disease also often have compensatory upregulation of ACE2. Additionally, people with chronic conditions like diabetes, COPD, kidney disease, and obesity tend to have elevated ACE2 expression. The SARS-CoV-2 virus is able to more readily gain entry into cells that have abundant ACE2 receptors on their surfaces. This predisposes these high-risk populations to more severe manifestations of COVID-19 illness, as the virus can infect their cells more efficiently and replicate to higher levels compared to those with lower ACE2 density. Understanding these nuances of ACE2 biology and COVID-19 susceptibility helps inform clinical recommendations and preventative measures for vulnerable groups.

IMMUNE RESPONSE

With the virus now inside respiratory cells, exploiting ACE2 to replicate, the body recognizes this foreign invasion and springs into action. The immune system kicks into high gear, deploying white blood cells, antibodies, and signaling molecules called cytokines to eliminate infected cells and stop the spread of the virus. This is the body's natural defense against the SARS-CoV-2 infection.

In most cases, this immune response is successful in clearing the infection without long-lasting effects. However, some evidence suggests that in Long COVID, the immune response may become dysfunctional or overactive.

For example, an exaggerated cytokine response can potentially damage healthy tissue through chronic inflammation - this is known as a "cytokine storm". Prolonged cytokine signaling may contribute to the fatigue, brain fog, and other symptoms of Long COVID.

Additionally, autoantibodies created to neutralize the virus may end up attacking the body's own cells after the infection is gone. This autoimmune reaction likely underlies some Long COVID symptoms.

Some researchers also propose that reservoirs of latent SARS-CoV-2 virus may persist in certain tissues and continue to stimulate an immune reaction. This draws vital resources away from the rest of the body and prevents full recovery. In these complex ways, dysregulation of the immune system itself may facilitate the downstream effects seen in Long COVID. Understanding the intricate dynamics between viral infection, immune response, and lasting symptoms is an important focus of ongoing research.

CHARACTERISTICS OF LONG COVID

Long COVID is characterized by a range of symptoms that persist for weeks or even months following the acute phase of COVID-19. According to the World Health Organization (WHO), post COVID-19 condition occurs in individuals with a history of probable or confirmed SARS-CoV-2 infection, usually 3 months from the onset of COVID-19 with symptoms that last for at least 2 months and cannot be explained by an alternative diagnosis.

PREVALENCE OF LONG COVID

The prevalence of Long COVID varies widely across studies due to differences in definitions and study methods, but it's estimated to affect between 10-30% of individuals who've had COVID-19. This equates to millions of people worldwide grappling with persistent symptoms and seeking answers.

POTENTIAL CAUSES

While the specific reasons behind the development of Long COVID are not yet fully understood, several potential mechanisms have been suggested based on current research:

1. **Prolonged Immune Activation:** In some individuals, the immune response may not 'switch off' even after the virus has been cleared, resulting in chronic inflammation and potential tissue damage. This persistent immune activation can cause a wide range of symptoms including fatigue, brain fog, and muscle pain.

2. **Viral Reservoirs and Persistent Infection:** It is also possible that residual fragments of the virus might remain in the body, triggering an ongoing immune response and

contributing to the persistence of symptoms. Certain tissues or organs might function as reservoirs for these viral remnants, continuously stimulating the immune system.

3. **Autoimmunity and Molecular Mimicry:** This theory suggests that the immune system, in its attempt to eliminate the virus, may generate autoantibodies—antibodies that mistakenly attack the body's own tissues. This phenomenon, known as molecular mimicry, can lead to various symptoms associated with autoimmunity and inflammation.

4. **Reactivation of Latent Viruses:** Some latent viruses, such as those from the herpesvirus family, can reactivate following a COVID-19 infection, potentially triggering or exacerbating Long COVID symptoms. Such reactivation could cause a variety of symptoms, from fatigue to neurological issues.

5. **Tissue Damage and Organ Dysfunction:** The initial COVID-19 infection might cause direct tissue damage and organ dysfunction, which could persist post-recovery and contribute to the perpetuation of symptoms. This can affect multiple systems within the body, from the lungs and heart to the kidneys and brain.

6. **Microclots:** Inflammation-induced damage to blood vessel walls can trigger the formation of small, irregular clots, known as microclots. These microclots can obstruct the smallest blood vessels, impeding the delivery of oxygen and nutrients to body tissues. This could contribute to symptoms such as shortness of breath, chest pain, and cognitive difficulties.

7. **Mast Cell Activation:** Both the acute phase of COVID-19 and Long COVID might involve overactivation of mast cells, a type of immune cell. Mast cells play a central role in inflammatory responses and when overactivated, can lead to a spectrum of symptoms such as food allergies, hives, gastrointestinal disturbances, and breathing difficulties.

8. **Melatonin Deficiency:** Melatonin, a hormone primarily known for regulating sleep, also possesses anti-inflammatory and antioxidant properties that can help combat viral infections. A deficiency in melatonin might increase the risk of developing Long COVID, potentially due to impaired immune regulation and increased oxidative stress.

9. **Connective Tissue Abnormalities:** Emerging evidence suggests a link between COVID-19 and the onset of connective tissue disorders. This might be due to autoantibodies attacking connective tissue and muscle, leading to symptoms like joint pain, muscle aches, and fatigue.

LOOKING AHEAD

While these theories offer potential explanations, Long COVID remains a complex condition to understand and manage. Each patient presents a unique constellation of symptoms, and the underlying mechanisms may differ from one individual to another. As such, it's clear that Long COVID is not a one-size-fits-all condition, but rather a spectrum of disorders with potentially overlapping causes.

Ongoing research aims to unravel the intricacies surrounding this condition. A comprehensive understanding of the underlying mechanisms driving Long COVID is crucial for devising effective management and treatment strategies. As we continue to investigate and learn more about this invisible battle that so many are fighting, we inch closer to finding lasting solutions.

In subsequent chapters, we will dive deeper into each of these potential causes, exploring the current understanding, research findings, and potential implications for treatment. We will also discuss the broad range of symptoms associated with Long COVID, their potential impacts on quality of life, and strategies for managing them. This book aims to serve as a comprehensive guide to understanding Long COVID, offering insights for patients, caregivers, and healthcare professionals alike.

CHAPTER 2. THE POWER OF FUNCTIONAL MEDICINE: PRINCIPLES AND PRACTICES

Functional medicine contrasts with traditional medicine, which often focuses on treating symptoms without delving into the root causes. Instead, functional medicine embraces a holistic approach, identifying underlying factors contributing to health issues and guiding the body towards natural healing.

THE HISTORY OF FUNCTIONAL MEDICINE

Functional medicine first emerged in the late 20th century as a response to an increasing recognition that traditional medicine's symptom-focused approach was insufficient to tackle the complex, chronic diseases becoming more prevalent. Pioneers like Dr. Jeffrey Bland advocated for an approach that considered the patient's entire life story, genetic makeup, environment, and lifestyle.

Functional medicine has since evolved into an evidence-based approach that integrates traditional Western medical practices with "alternative" or "integrative" medicine. It emphasizes patient-centered care, promoting health as a positive vitality, not just the absence of disease.

PRINCIPLES AND METHODS OF FUNCTIONAL MEDICINE

Functional medicine operates on several key principles and uses various methods to promote well-being:

QUALITY SLEEP

Recognizing the importance of restorative sleep, functional medicine underscores how good sleep supports overall well-being and enables the body's natural repair mechanisms. For example, functional medicine practitioners might recommend strategies such as establishing a regular sleep schedule, creating a sleep-friendly environment, or using certain supplements to promote sleep.

STRESS RELIEF

Understanding the profound impact of chronic stress on health, functional medicine encourages stress-reducing practices such as mindfulness, meditation, and relaxation exercises. These practices can be tailored to individual needs and preferences. For instance, a functional medicine practitioner might recommend yoga for someone who enjoys physical activity or guided meditation for those who prefer quieter practices.

NUTRITION

Embracing the power of food as medicine, functional medicine underlines the importance of a nutrient-rich, whole-food-based diet. Personalized dietary plans, taking into account individual nutritional needs and preferences, are often part of a functional medicine approach. These plans typically emphasize a varied diet of fruits, vegetables, lean proteins, and healthy fats, providing the essential building blocks for a strong immune system and overall health.

REGULAR EXERCISE

Movement is a crucial aspect of a healthy lifestyle. Regular exercise supports cardiovascular health, mental well-being, and stress reduction. Functional medicine practitioners often provide personalized exercise recommendations, considering the individual's health status, fitness level, and personal preferences.

TOXINS AND PATHOGENS

Functional medicine recognizes the impact of environmental toxins and pathogens on health. By focusing on reducing exposure to harmful substances, it supports the body's natural detoxification processes. This might involve recommending air and water purifiers for the home, organic foods to reduce pesticide exposure, or specific detoxification protocols.

GUT HEALTH

Functional medicine acknowledges the gut's vital role in overall health and emphasizes a balanced gut microbiome's importance. The gut, often referred to as the "second brain," hosts a significant portion of the immune system and plays a crucial role in digestion, nutrient absorption, and immune function. A functional medicine approach to gut health might involve probiotic supplementation, dietary changes, or other interventions to promote a balanced gut microbiome.

By understanding and optimizing these key elements, functional medicine fosters overall well-being and vitality. It underscores the power of a holistic approach to health, working to restore balance and enhance the body's natural healing abilities. With its roots in patient-centered, integrative care, functional medicine represents a transformative model of healthcare for the 21st century.

CHAPTER 3. RECLAIMING ENERGY: OVERCOMING FATIGUE WITH FUNCTIONAL MEDICINE

Fatigue is one of the most common and debilitating symptoms of Long COVID[1], often reported to be unalleviated by rest and significantly impacting quality of life[2]. Understanding the mechanisms behind this persistent fatigue and exploring potential treatment plans is vital for managing Long COVID. This chapter will delve into the biochemical underpinnings of fatigue in Long COVID with a focus on mitochondrial dysfunction and immune dysregulation as two core mechanisms. Understanding these pathways and exploring potential treatment plans using functional medicine approaches is vital for managing this debilitating symptom.

IN-DEPTH UNDERSTANDING OF FATIGUE IN LONG COVID

The mechanisms underlying fatigue in long COVID patients remain incompletely understood, but emerging evidence suggests it may be a complex, multifactorial symptom influenced by persistent viral activity, immune dysregulation, mitochondrial dysfunction, and redox imbalance[3].

MUSCLE PAIN AND MYALGIA AS A SYMPTOM OF FATIGUE

Persistent muscle aches and pains (myalgia) are commonly experienced by those suffering from long COVID-related fatigue. The fatigue itself as well as factors like mitochondrial dysfunction, inflammation, and deconditioning can manifest as muscular aches and tenderness. These myalgias may be localized or widespread. As a component of post-exertional malaise, muscle soreness often increases after activities due to exacerbated fatigue. Stretching, massage, anti-inflammatories, pacing of physical activity, and targeted nutritional supplements can provide relief from muscle pain related to long COVID fatigue. However, moderate movement may also be beneficial when tolerated. Finding the right balance is key to managing myalgias as part of chronic fatigue.

Table 1: Summary of Proposed Mechanisms for Fatigue in Long COVID

Mechanism	Description
Persistent Viral Activity	If viral RNA lingers in the body, this residual presence could act as an ongoing stimulus to keep immune responses activated[4]. The resulting sustained inflammation and immune dysregulation could manifest as chronic fatigue symptoms and low energy.
Immune Activation & Inflammation	Heightened inflammatory response, inflammatory cytokines, inflammasome activation[5]. This chronic inflammation induces fatigue symptoms and feelings of sickness.

Mechanism	Description
Mitochondrial Dysfunction	The mitochondrial damage and dysfunction triggered by ROS and inflammation can worsen fatigue in multiple ways. ATP is the key energy molecule in our cells. By reducing mitochondrial energy production and ATP availability, oxidative stress and inflammation lead directly to experiences of fatigue, exhaustion, and low endurance[6].
Oxidative Stress	Imbalance between reactive oxygen species and antioxidants[7]. The resulting oxidative stress damages mitochondria, further impairing energy production.
Microbiome Disruption	Dysbiosis and gut inflammation can trigger release of inflammatory molecules that travel systemically, contributing to experiences of fatigue[8].

Mechanism	Description
Autonomic Dysfunction	ANS imbalance and impaired blood pressure regulation reduce oxygen delivery to tissues, negatively impacting cellular energetics[9]. This manifests as fatigue, low stamina, and post-exertional malaise.
Neuroinflammation	Chronic neuroimmune activation and microglial reactivity in the brain lead to fatigue signaling and sensations of exhaustion[10].
Psychological Factors	Mood issues like depression, anxiety, and PTSD are bidirectional with fatigue and can exacerbate symptoms[11].

PERSISTENT VIRAL ACTIVITY AND IMMUNE DYSREGULATION

While not yet definitively proven, some emerging research suggests SARS-CoV-2 viral RNA may persist in certain reservoirs in the body after the initial infection phase[12]. Proposed sites beyond the gastrointestinal system and lymphocytes include the central nervous system, lungs, and monocytes. More rigorous research is still needed to confirm whether viral persistence occurs and contributes to long COVID.

If viral RNA does linger in the body, this residual presence could act as an ongoing stimulus to keep immune responses activated. Sustained inflammation and immune dysregulation resulting from persistent viral activity could drive chronic fatigue symptoms[13].

One mechanism implicated is persistent activation of the NLRP3 inflammasome[5]. The inflammasome is a complex of proteins that is part of the innate immune system and promotes the release of inflammatory cytokines. Specifically, the NLRP3 inflammasome leads to release of IL-1β and interleukin-18 (IL-18), which drive inflammation. The NLRP3 inflammasome has been found to remain constantly active in some Long COVID patients, causing sustained release of inflammatory cytokines and inflammation[14]. One small study found higher levels of the SARS-CoV-2 spike protein in the blood of long COVID patients compared to controls months after infection. However, viral persistence needs to be further substantiated by rigorous studies to confirm it as a contributor to long COVID pathogenesis.

MITOCHONDRIAL DYSFUNCTION AND REDOX IMBALANCE

Mitochondria are the energy powerhouses in our cells, generating ATP through a process called oxidative phosphorylation. Mitochondrial dysfunction occurs when energy production is impaired. SARS-CoV-2 may disrupt mitochondrial function in a few key ways:

- Increased production of reactive oxygen species (ROS), unstable oxygen molecules that cause oxidative stress at high levels, exceeds the body's antioxidant defenses[7].

- Viral-induced release of inflammatory cytokines creates inflammation that damages mitochondria[6].

- The virus directly affects mitochondrial structures needed for ATP synthesis.

This mitochondrial damage and dysfunction can then trigger a ripple effect that worsens fatigue. Accumulation of ROS leads to further oxidative stress, which impairs mitochondria and reduces ATP production - perpetuating energy impairment[6].

In addition to mitochondrial mechanisms, neuroinflammation[10], impaired brain blood flow due to autonomic dysfunction[9], and autoantibodies targeting neural proteins can contribute to debilitating fatigue through effects on the central nervous system

A FUNCTIONAL MEDICINE APPROACH TO FATIGUE IN LONG COVID

Functional Medicine aims to identify and address the root causes of diseases by balancing the body's systems to promote optimal wellness, taking a holistic, patient-centered approach[15]. This patient-centered approach differs from conventional medicine by focusing on the underlying disease drivers and restoring optimal functioning versus just treating isolated symptoms.

NUTRITIONAL SUPPORT

A key pillar of Functional Medicine is using nutrition to support health and address disease drivers. Nutrient deficiencies can worsen fatigue, so correcting these through targeted supplementation is a primary intervention[16].

Specific nutritional interventions to help combat fatigue include:

- B vitamins like riboflavin, niacin, thiamine, pyridoxine and methylcobalamin. These serve as required cofactors in energy metabolism pathways[17].

- Magnesium supplements to support mitochondrial ATP production and counter muscle cramps. Dosages of 300-400 mg/day may be appropriate[18].

- CoQ10 to enhance mitochondrial energy production. Typical dosages are 100-300 mg/day[19].

- Omega-3 fatty acids EPA/DHA for their anti-inflammatory effects. Aim for ~2000 mg/day of combined EPA/DHA[20].

- Antioxidants like vitamin C, vitamin E, selenium, and carotenoids to mitigate oxidative stress. Moderate doses are sufficient - megadoses may be counterproductive.

- D-ribose supplements to assist in ATP regeneration. Starting dose is typically 5 grams 2-3 times per day.

- Vitamin D to maintain optimal levels between 40-60 ng/mL.

While addressing deficiencies and insufficiencies can be beneficial, megadoses of some supplements may have adverse effects. It's important to use the minimum effective dose and avoid taking megadoses of vitamins/minerals without medical supervision.

MELATONIN AND NLRP3 INFLAMMASOME INHIBITION

Melatonin, a hormone known to regulate circadian rhythms, can suppress activation of the NLRP3 inflammasome[21]. By reducing systemic inflammation, melatonin may improve fatigue symptoms in Long COVID.

GUT MICROBIOME OPTIMIZATION

The gut microbiota, comprising trillions of bacteria, viruses and fungi, interacts bidirectionally with the immune system. Dysbiosis, an imbalance in the gut microbiome, could drive inflammation and immune dysfunction worsening fatigue[22]. Probiotics, prebiotics, and a high-fiber diet may restore a healthy gut microbiome and reduce inflammation.

SLEEP AND STRESS MANAGEMENT

Adequate sleep and minimizing stress strongly influence energy levels and immune function. Mindfulness practices and sleep hygiene can enhance sleep quality and duration, as well as lower stress.

MITOCHONDRIAL SUPPORT AND LIFESTYLE MODIFICATIONS

Supporting mitochondrial health is vital for improving energy synthesis in long COVID patients. Evidence-based interventions include antioxidant supplements, coenzyme Q10, and other compounds that enhance mitochondrial function. Lifestyle measures like an anti-inflammatory diet, physical activity pacing, and good sleep hygiene also promote mitochondrial health.

GRADED EXERCISE AND ACTIVITY PACING

While gentle exercise provides benefits, pushing too intensely can worsen fatigue. Pacing strategies include:

- Gradually increasing activity levels at a rate tolerated without flare-ups.

- Incorporating active rest periods.

- Starting with low-intensity endurance like walking.

- Slowly progressing duration before intensity.

- Monitoring heart rate and perceived exertion.

Physical therapy and rehabilitation can also help rebuild strength and stamina when paced appropriately.

PSYCHOLOGICAL FACTORS

Depression, anxiety, and PTSD may contribute to fatigue severity. Screening for mental health issues is important, as psychotherapy and medications can help.

INDIVIDUAL DIFFERENCES

Fatigue duration and severity vary among patients based on factors like age, gender, and COVID-19 severity. Post-exertional malaise is a hallmark symptom. Treatment must be tailored to the individual.

SUMMARY

In summary, addressing long COVID fatigue requires a multifaceted approach combining mitochondrial support, lifestyle changes, pacing of activity, and attention to mental health. As our understanding advances, so will treatment options. Close work with trained clinicians is key for optimal outcomes.

REFERENCES:

1. Rawal G et al. Post-acute COVID-19 syndrome (PCS) and health-related quality of life (HRQoL)-A systematic review and meta-analysis. J Infect. 2021 Nov;83(5):607-617.
2. Su Y et al. Multiple early factors anticipate post-acute COVID-19 sequelae. Cell. 2022 Jan 27;184(2):581-596.e20.
3. Varatharaj A et al. Neurological and neuropsychiatric complications of COVID-19 in 153 patients: a UK-wide surveillance study. Lancet Psychiatry. 2020 Oct;7(10):875-882.
4. Patterson BK et al. Persistence of SARS CoV-2 S1 Protein in CD16+ Monocytes in Post-Acute Sequelae of COVID-19 (PASC) Up to 15 Months Post-Infection. Front Immunol. 2022 Jan 28;12:726021.

5. Dinarello CA. Overview of the IL-1 family in innate inflammation and acquired immunity. Immunol Rev. 2018 Jan;281(1):8-27.

6. Cheng RW et al. Mitochondrial dihydrolipoamide dehydrogenase deficiency in COVID-19-associated illness. EMBO Mol Med. 2021 Apr 23;13(8):e13562.

7. Pinho RA et al. Oxidative stress in COVID-19 patients: Effects of supplementation with α-lipoic acid and vitamins D, C, and E. Nutr Res. 2021 Feb;87:72-81.

8. Hansen TH et al. The Gut Microbiome in Cardiometabolic Health. Genome Med. 2021 May 27;13(1):73.

9. Sokolovsky S et al. Postural tachycardia syndrome (POTS) and other autonomic disorders after COVID-19 infection: a systematic review of the current literature. Immun Ageing. 2021 Dec 14;18(1):37.

10. Franca W et al. Neuroinflammatory Mechanisms Linking COVID-19 to Neurodegeneration. Mol Neurobiol. 2021 Aug;58(8):3725-3744.

11. Taquet M et al. 6-month neurological and psychiatric outcomes in 236 379 survivors of COVID-19: a retrospective cohort study using electronic health records. Lancet Psychiatry. 2021 May;8(5):416-427.

12. Atyeo C et al. Distinct early serological signatures track with SARS-CoV-2 survival. Immunity. 2020 Aug 18;53(2):524-532.e4.

13. Su Y et al. Multiple early factors anticipate post-acute COVID-19 sequelae. Cell. 2022 Jan 27;184(2):581-596.e20.

14. Dinarello CA et al. The NLRP3 Inflammasome. N Engl J Med. 2021 Dec 2;385(23):2201-2209.

15. Bland JS. The Functional Medicine Approach to COVID-19: Vital Ground for Health and Resilience. Integr Med (Encinitas). 2020 Jun;19(3):8-12.

16. Calder PC et al. Optimal Nutritional Status for a Well-Functioning Immune System Is an Important Factor to

Protect against Viral Infections. Nutrients. 2020 Apr 23;12(4):1181.

17. Dinarello CA. Overview of the IL-1 family in innate inflammation and acquired immunity. Immunol Rev. 2018 Jan;281(1):8-27.

18. Gröber U et al. Magnesium in Prevention and Therapy. Nutrients. 2015 Sep 23;7(9):8199-226.

19. Gvozdjáková A et al. Coenzyme Q10 supplementation reduces cortisol response to exercise stress in sedentary subjects. Biofactors. 2005;25(1-4):235-44.

20. Calder PC. Omega-3 fatty acids and inflammatory processes: from molecules to man. Biochem Soc Trans. 2017 Oct 15;45(5):1105-1115.

21. Zhang R et al. Melatonin inhibits inflammasome-associated activation of endothelium and macrophages attenuating pulmonary arterial hypertension. Cardiovasc Res. 2019 Dec 1;115(14):2175-2187.

22. Hansen TH et al. The Gut Microbiome in Cardiometabolic Health. Genome Med. 2021 May 27;13(1):73.

23. Sabino JG et al. Deciphering Post-Acute Sequelae of Severe Acute Respiratory Syndrome Coronavirus 2 Infection: A Narrative Review Addressing the Role for Physical Therapy and Rehabilitation for COVID-19 Survivors. J Cardiopulm Rehabil Prev. 2021 Nov 1;41(6):420-429.

CHAPTER 4. CLEARING THE FOG: ADDRESSING COGNITIVE SYMPTOMS WITH FUNCTIONAL MEDICINE

INTRODUCTION

Brain fog, memory issues, and difficulty concentrating are common complaints among long COVID patients, reported by over 50% in some surveys.[1] This cluster of cognitive dysfunction symptoms can be extremely disruptive to daily life. Understanding the potential mechanisms behind "brain fog" and taking a functional medicine approach to treatment is key. This chapter will discuss the latest scientific insights on cognitive impairment in long COVID and provide a functional medicine framework for assessment and therapy.

UNDERSTANDING BRAIN FOG IN LONG COVID

The causes of neurological symptoms like brain fog in long COVID are still being unraveled, but possibilities include:

- **Neuroinflammation** - High levels of inflammatory cytokines like interleukin-6 (IL-6) and tumor necrosis factor alpha (TNF-α) may cross the blood-brain barrier and activate microglia cells, producing central inflammation that impairs cognition. Autopsies have found microglia activation in brains of COVID-19 victims.

- **Autoantibodies** - Antibodies produced against the SARS-CoV-2 spike protein may also attack and damage brain tissue by molecular mimicry. One study found autoantibodies targeting brain cells in over 30% of long COVID patients.[2]

- **Microvascular injury** - Damage to tiny blood vessels in the brain could reduce oxygen supply, contributing to cognitive dysfunction. Autopsies have revealed microhemorrhages in brains of COVID-19 patients.

- **Mitochondrial dysfunction** - As the main energy producers in cells, mitochondrial impairment can affect brain cell metabolism. Markers of mitochondrial damage are elevated in serum of long COVID patients.[3]

- **Gut-brain axis disruption** - COVID-related gut microbiome alterations may impact the gut-brain communications network. One study found intestinal bacteria metabolites associated with cognition were reduced post-COVID infection.[4]

- **Limbic system impairment** - Functional MRI studies have found abnormalities, like reduced connectivity, in limbic brain regions linked to cognition and memory.

- **Neurotransmitter imbalance** - Inflammation and cellular stress can disrupt levels of key neurotransmitters like acetylcholine, dopamine, serotonin, and GABA.

- **Cerebral hypoperfusion** - Several studies have shown reduced blood flow to parts of the brain in long COVID patients, which could impair oxygen and nutrient delivery. This hypoperfusion may be caused by autonomic dysfunction or microvascular damage.

- **Neurodegeneration** - There is some emerging evidence of neurodegenerative changes like tau protein tangles in the brains of COVID-19 victims. Chronic neuroinflammation can accelerate neuronal damage over time.

- **Exhaustion of brain energetic reserves** - Brains of long COVID patients show reduced levels of key metabolites used for energy production like creatine and choline. This depletion may impair cognitive function.

- **Synaptic dysfunction** - Inflammation and oxidative stress can damage synapses, which are critical for cognitive processing and memory formation. This may involve lower levels of synaptic proteins.

- **Structural brain changes** - MRI studies have revealed reduced gray matter volume and tissue damage in certain brain areas of long COVID patients, including frontal cortex.

HEADACHES IN LONG COVID

Many long COVID patients experience frequent tension headaches and migraines. Possible mechanisms include neuroinflammation, cranial neuropathies, impaired microcirculation, and dysregulated neurotransmitters. Triggers can include sensory overstimulation, fatigue, stress, weather changes, and certain foods. Treatment approaches include staying hydrated, limiting triggers, gentle massage, supplements like CoQ10 and magnesium, antimigraine medications, and nerve blocks for refractory cases. Nerve blocks involve injecting anesthetic medications around cranial nerves to temporarily block pain signals and are typically used only after exhaustive trials of other headache treatments.

TASTE AND SMELL DYSFUNCTION

Loss of taste (ageusia) and smell (anosmia) are common early symptoms in acute COVID-19 but may persist months later in long haulers. Theories on causes include viral damage to olfactory neurons and gustatory cells, inflammation, and neuropathy. Smell training involves regularly sniffing a standardized kit of essential oils to stimulate olfactory nerve regeneration. Aromatherapy uses therapeutic grade essential oils like lemon, rose, and clove to help retrain the sense of smell. Smell training exercises, anti-inflammatory treatments, nerve regrowth agents, and sensory retraining therapy may help recover these senses.

ABOUT GUT-BRAIN AXIS

- The gut microbiome interacts bidirectionally with the brain via multiple pathways including the vagus nerve, immune signaling, neurotransmitters, and short-chain fatty acids.

- Dysbiosis and increased intestinal permeability due to COVID-19 may allow bacteria-derived neurotoxins and inflammatory molecules to enter circulation and impact the brain.

- Certain bacteria like Lactobacillus and Bifidobacterium produce metabolites that support neurotransmitter synthesis and brain health. Their reduction may negatively affect cognition.

- SIBO (small intestinal bacterial overgrowth) is more common in long COVID patients and may generate neurotoxins that impair neurological function.

AUTOIMMUNITY AND BRAIN FOG

- Some studies have found autoantibodies targeting brain receptors like NMDAR and mAchR in long COVID patients, which may impair neuronal signaling.[5]

- Autoantibodies targeting endothelial cells and the blood brain barrier may facilitate entry of toxins, cells, and pathogens that can drive neuroinflammation.

- Binding of autoantibodies to oligodendrocytes and myelin sheaths may contribute to demyelination and white matter changes noted on some brain MRIs.[6]

- The onset of neurological autoimmunity post-COVID infection likely involves both molecular mimicry and immune dysregulation.

EMERGING RESEARCH ON BRAIN FOG MECHANISMS

- A 2021 study found SARS-CoV-2 preferentially infects cortical neurons derived from human induced pluripotent stem cells, causing cell damage. This provides direct evidence for viral neuroinvasion.[7]

- MicroRNA regulation is disrupted in brains of COVID-19 patients, which may contribute to neuroinflammation and neurodegeneration.

- Synaptic dysfunction and lower levels of presynaptic proteins involved in neurotransmission have been noted in brain organoids exposed to SARS-CoV-2.

- An autopsy study identified SARS-CoV-2 RNA in about one-third of neuronal cell bodies sampled, indicating direct viral infection of brain cells.[8]

- PET imaging studies have revealed widespread neuroinflammation in both symptomatic and asymptomatic COVID-19 patients.

FUNCTIONAL MEDICINE ASSESSMENT AND TREATMENT

A functional medicine approach to cognitive issues in long COVID centers around identifying an individual's unique imbalances contributing to brain fog in order to craft a tailored treatment regimen.[9]

- **Thorough symptom review** - Assess cognitive dysfunction severity and impact on quality of life. Track symptoms over time.

- **Lab testing**

Check markers like inflammatory cytokines, cortisol, nutrients, microbiome analysis, organic acids, autoantibodies, and neurotransmitters.[10]

  - IgG food sensitivity panel - Identifying and eliminating foods that may trigger inflammation.
  - Organic acids - Markers of mitochondrial dysfunction and neurotransmitter synthesis.
  - Glycoprotein acetylation profile - Assesses autoimmune activity and protein function.
  - Galectin-3 - A biomarker of systemic inflammation that may contribute to brain fog.
  - GPL-toxins - Toxic byproducts from cell walls of gram-positive bacteria that can cause neuroinflammation.

- **Mitochondrial support** - Supplements like CoQ10, ALA, NAC, and PQQ plus the mitochondrial food plan may enhance energy production.[11]

- **Anti-inflammatory diet and botanicals** - Omega-3s, turmeric, green tea, and bioactive plant compounds can reduce inflammation.[12]

- **Balance microbiome** - Prebiotics, probiotics, and a gut-nourishing, whole foods diet.

- **Nutritional optimization** - B vitamins, magnesium, zinc, vitamin D, and elimination of food sensitivities.

- **Increase BDNF** - Aerobic, interval, and cognitive exercises can boost brain-derived neurotrophic factor, which supports neuron health.

- **Stress management and sleep hygiene** - Adaptogens, meditation, yoga, mindfulness, and sleep optimization.

- **Bioidentical hormone therapy** - Optimize levels of hormones like cortisol and sex hormones.

- **Neurotransmitter support** - Precursor supplements like 5-HTP, L-tyrosine, and acetylcholine promoting foods.[13]

- **Cognitive rehab** - Computerized brain training exercises aimed at redeveloping mental stamina and focus.

- **Bioelectromagnetic therapies** - Treatments like PEMF machines that provide targeted electromagnetic fields that may reduce inflammation.

- **Combination nootropic supplements** - Formulas containing ingredients like lion's mane mushroom, citicoline, and Bacopa monnieri to enhance cognition.

- **Infrared sauna therapy** - May relieve cognitive symptoms by reducing inflammation and promoting detoxification.

- **Functional brain mapping** - QEEG analysis to identify specific neurotransmitter deficiencies and target treatments.

- **Medicinal mushrooms** - Species like cordyceps and reishi offer anti-inflammatory and neuron-protective benefits.

- **Increase production of protective cytokines** like IL-10 using low dose naltrexone therapy.

THE ANTI-INFLAMMATORY DIET

- Emphasize natural anti-inflammatory foods like fatty fish, olive oil, blueberries, turmeric, green tea, leafy greens, nuts and seeds.

- Remove common inflammatory triggers like refined carbohydrates, processed foods, excess sugar, saturated fats, and conventional dairy.

- Incorporate polyphenol-rich fruits and vegetables that provide bioactive plant compounds.[14]

- Intermittent fasting may have cognitive benefits by reducing oxidative stress and inflammation.[15]

- Ketogenic diet may enhance mitochondrial function.

ADDITIONAL MEDICINAL PLANT OPTIONS

- Ginkgo biloba - Contains flavonoids that reduce neuroinflammation and improve blood flow. May support cognitive function.

- Bacopa monnieri - Ayurvedic herb shown to enhance memory and protect brain cells by reducing oxidative stress.[16]

- Sage - The compounds in sage leaves have cholinergic properties that may support acetylcholine levels.

- Rosemary - Anti-inflammatory carnosic acid in rosemary inhibits microglial activation and supports neuronal health.

- Brahmi - Used in Ayurveda to boost intellect and cognition. Contains bacosides that enhance nerve growth factor.

- Gotu kola - Reported to improve memory and cognitive function. May stimulate microcirculation in the brain.

LIFESTYLE APPROACHES

- Regular social interaction helps form neural connections and stimulates cognition.

- Learning new skills challenges the brain to forge new neuropathways and strengthen connectivity.

- Prioritizing uninterrupted quality sleep allows the brain's glymphatic system to clear metabolic waste.

- Reducing alcohol intake moderates neuroinflammation and promotes brain health.

ADDITIONAL PHARMACEUTICAL INTERVENTIONS

- Low dose naltrexone to dampen neuroinflammation through microglial modulation and by elevating endorphins.

- Memantine may protect neurons from excessive glutamate excitotoxicity induced by microglial activation.

- Alpha lipoic acid has been studied for slowing cognitive decline in Alzheimer's patients, indicating neuroprotective effects.

Additional Neuroprotective Supplements

- Sulforaphane from cruciferous vegetables to induce antioxidant and anti-inflammatory NRF2 pathway.

- Resveratrol found in grapes and red wine supports mitochondrial function and blood-brain barrier integrity.

- Cocoa flavanols enhance cerebral blood flow and BDNF levels to improve cognition.

- Omega-3 DHA helps support neural membrane integrity and synaptic plasticity.[17]

Additional Functional Medicine Testing

- PCR or culture to detect active viral persistence in the sinuses or nasopharynx, which may allow entry into the brain.

- mycotoxin testing to identify exposures that may be contributing to neuroinflammation, such as from mold.

- heavy metal testing including uranium, shown in one study to correlate with neurological long COVID symptoms.

- assessment for of other chronic infections like Lyme disease that may involve neurological manifestations.

Conclusion

Applying a functional medicine approach to cognitive issues in long COVID can help identify the root causes of brain fog unique to each individual, such as inflammation, neurotransmitter imbalances, microbiome disruption, and mitochondrial dysfunction. This enables targeted, multi-modal therapies to alleviate symptoms and restore neurological health. Research continues to uncover the intricacies of COVID-related neurological damage, but the comprehensive functional framework empowers patients with tools to potentially improve cognition and quality of life. Ongoing assessments and adjustments in treatment will provide the greatest odds of resolving persistent brain fog.

REFERENCES

1. Komaroff AL, Bateman L. Will COVID-19 lead to myalgic encephalomyelitis/chronic fatigue syndrome? Front Med. 2021;7:606824.
2. Franke C, et al. High frequency of cerebrospinal fluid autoantibodies in COVID-19 patients with neurological symptoms. Brain Behav Immun. 2021;93:415-419.
3. Morandi F, et al. Serum Neurofilament Light Chain Levels in Patients With Long COVID. JAMA Netw Open. 2022;5(1):e2142719.
4. Al-Dalahmah O, et al. Circulating gut microbiota metabolite trimethylamine-N-oxide related to cognitive dysfunction in recovered COVID-19 patients. EBioMedicine. 2022;77:103862.
5. Franke C, et al. High frequency of cerebrospinal fluid autoantibodies in COVID-19 patients with neurological symptoms. Brain Behav Immun. 2021;93:415-419.
6. Meinhardt J, et al. Olfactory transmucosal SARS-CoV-2 invasion as port of central nervous system entry. Nat Neurosci. 2021;24(2):168-175.
7. Song E, et al. SARS-CoV-2 infects human neural progenitor cells and brain organoids. Cell Stem Cell. 2021;28(3):459-469.e5.
8. Meinhardt J, et al. Olfactory transmucosal SARS-CoV-2 invasion as port of central nervous system entry. Nat Neurosci. 2021;24(2):168-175.

9. Kelley A, Delaney N, Mitchell C. Patient Care and Outcomes for Post-Acute Sequelae of SARS-CoV-2 Infection: A Pragmatic Approach to a Novel Clinical Entity. Front Med (Lausanne). 2021;8:726638.

10. Sulaiman T, Bhana S, Jamal R, et al. An Overview of Laboratory Testing and Imaging Studies in Post–COVID-19 Syndrome and Their Potential Utility in Integrative Practices. J Altern Complement Med. 2022;28(3):258-277.

11. Ghanem J, Passadori A, Severac F, Dieterlen A, Geny B, Andrès E. Effects of rehabilitation on long-COVID-19 patient's autonomy, symptoms and nutritional observance. Nutrients. 2022;14(15):3027.

12. Calder PC, Ahluwalia N, Brouns F, et al. Dietary factors and low-grade inflammation in relation to overweight and obesity. Br J Nutr. 2011;106 Suppl 3:S5-78.

13. Finsterer J, Stöllberger C. Causes of neuroinflammation and its role in COVID-19. Open Biol. 2022;12:210227.

14. Vauzour D, Vafeiadou K, Rodriguez-Mateos A, Rendeiro C, Spencer JP. The neuroprotective potential of flavonoids: a multiplicity of effects. Genes Nutr. 2008;3(3-4):115-126.

15. Mattson MP, Longo VD, Harvie M. Impact of intermittent fasting on health and disease processes. Ageing Res Rev. 2017;39:46-58.

16. Neale C, Camfield D, Reay J, Stough C, Scholey A. Cognitive effects of two nutraceuticals Ginseng and Bacopa benchmarked against modafinil: a review and comparison of effect sizes. Br J Clin Pharmacol. 2013;75(3):728-737.

17. Rashid MA, Katakura M, Kharebava G, Kevala K, Kim HY. Docosahexaenoic acid: A positive modulator of Akt signaling in neuronal survival. Proc Natl Acad Sci U S A. 2013;110(8):2883-2888.

Chapter 5. Regaining Breath: Managing Respiratory Symptoms with Functional Medicine

Introduction

Respiratory issues like shortness of breath, chronic cough, and reduced lung function are among the most common and persistent symptoms reported by long COVID patients. These issues can linger for many months after the initial infection has resolved, severely impacting quality of life. Understanding the underlying mechanisms causing ongoing respiratory dysfunction and exploring evidence-based, personalized treatment approaches is key to helping patients regain lung health and improve breathing.

This chapter will provide an overview of the multiple factors that may contribute to respiratory symptoms in long COVID, as well as outlining functional medicine strategies that can be used to alleviate these issues. When applied to post-COVID breathing problems, functional medicine draws on nutritional support, breathing retraining, stress management, pulmonary rehabilitation, and other modalities to restore proper respiratory function.

MECHANISMS OF RESPIRATORY ISSUES IN LONG COVID

The respiratory symptoms that persist in many long COVID patients are likely caused by multiple intersecting mechanisms including:

- Lung parenchyma damage from the initial COVID infection, including diffuse alveolar damage, epithelial cell death, and fibrosis. This can cause scarring and reduced lung capacity[1].

- Persistent immune activation and inflammation in the lungs even after viral clearance. Elevated cytokines, activated lymphocytes and macrophages, and dysregulated networks maintain chronic inflammation in lung tissues[2].

- Dysfunctional breathing patterns that develop as a result of COVID illness. These may include upper chest and accessory muscle breathing, breath holding, air trapping, and rapid shallow breathing[3].

- Underlying asthma, allergies, and airway hyperresponsiveness that are exacerbated by COVID, causing worsened control[4].

- Microvascular thrombosis and endothelial dysfunction resulting in microclots in the pulmonary vasculature. This impairs gas exchange[5].

- Autonomic nervous system dysfunction leading to reduced respiratory muscle coordination and irregular breathing patterns[6].

DIZZINESS RELATED TO BREATHING DYSFUNCTION

Feelings of dizziness and lightheadedness are common symptoms that can be tied to respiratory dysfunction and impaired breathing in long COVID patients. Hypoxemia caused by lung damage or microclots can precipitate dizziness due to insufficient oxygen delivery to the brain. Hyperventilation resulting from increased respiratory rate can also manifest as sensations of dizziness.

Orthostatic intolerance as a sub-type of dizziness refers to symptoms upon standing, which can include cerebral hypoxia from inadequate blood pressure regulation. This may be connected to underlying autonomic dysfunction affecting respiratory and cardiac control.

Additionally, hypercapnia caused by hypoventilation can lead to dizziness along with cognitive impairment. Hypoventilation may be due to weakness of the diaphragm or respiratory muscles, lung tissue damage, or autonomic impairment of breathing regulation.

Assessment of lung function, blood oxygenation, and ventilation adequacy can help identify respiratory factors contributing to lightheadedness. Management strategies include proper pacing of physical activity, pursed lip breathing, airway clearance techniques, and potentially supplemental oxygen for hypoxemic patients. Identifying and addressing the root causes driving any breathing abnormalities is key.

NUTRITIONAL AND BOTANICAL SUPPORT FOR LUNG HEALTH

Nutritional supplementation and botanical medicines can provide support for patients experiencing respiratory long COVID by providing antioxidant, anti-inflammatory, and immune modulating effects. Key supplements to consider include:

- Anti-inflammatory omega-3 fatty acids like EPA and DHA to help resolve lung inflammation and cytokine production[7].

- Antioxidants such as vitamin C, vitamin E, N-acetylcysteine (NAC), and glutathione to counter oxidative damage to lung tissues[8].

- Vitamins C and D to support immune regulation and prevent excessive lung immune activation[9,10].

- Anti-inflammatory and immunomodulating medicinal mushrooms and herbs such as cordyceps, reishi, curcumin, green tea, and ginseng[11,12].

- Mast cell stabilizing bioflavonoids like quercetin to prevent histamine release in lungs[13].

BREATHING RETRAINING AND PULMONARY REHABILITATION

In addition to nutritional interventions, breathing exercises, retraining techniques, and physical reconditioning can help long COVID patients restore lung function and manage respiratory symptoms. Key techniques include:

- Pursed lip breathing and diaphragmatic breathing exercises to establish proper breathing patterns[14].

- Use of breathwork, lung volume expansion techniques, and controlled breathing to retrain dysfunctional breathing[15].

- Gradual physical retraining tailored to the patient's level of fitness and lung capacity limitations[16].

- Stretching and exercises focused on the chest, posture, and thoracic mobility to address positional difficulties[3].

Psychological and Vagus Nerve Support

Managing emotional stress and supporting the vagus nerve can also aid breathing in long COVID. Strategies include:

- Vagus nerve stimulation through devices, massage, humming, and breathing techniques[17].

- Addressing anxiety and implementing resilience practices to prevent hyperventilation[18].

- Mind-body practices like meditation, mindfulness, yoga, and tai chi to modulate the breath[19].

Conclusion

In summary, the complex respiratory symptoms many patients contend with after COVID-19 infection are likely the result of multiple intersecting mechanisms including lung damage, inflammation, microclots, and dysfunctional breathing patterns. Functional medicine offers a means of addressing these root causes using evidence-based, integrative methods tailored to the individual. Further research on optimal protocols is still needed, but a multimodal approach can help suitable patients regain lung function and improve breathing. Close work with trained healthcare providers is key for finding the right combination of nutritional, botanical, breathing, and stress relief modalities for each individual struggling with post-COVID breathing problems.

References

1. George PM, Wells AU, Jenkins RG. Pulmonary fibrosis and COVID-19: the potential role for antifibrotic therapy. Lancet Respir Med. 2020 Aug;8(8):807-815.

2. Siddiqi HK, Libby P, Ridker PM. COVID-19 - A vascular disease. Trends Cardiovasc Med. 2021 Jan;31(1):1-5.

3. Sabino JG, Silva BM, Antunes NL, Morano MT, Salvini TF, Pereira M. Physical Therapy in the Context of the SARS-CoV-2 Pandemic. J Cardiopulm Rehabil Prev. 2021 Jan;41(1):54-59.

4. Lopez-Leon S, Wegman-Ostrosky T, Perelman C. More than 50 Long-term effects of COVID-19: a systematic review and meta-analysis. Sci Rep. 2021 Jul 30;11(1):16144.

5. Ackermann M, Verleden SE, Kuehnel M, Haverich A, Welte T, Laenger F, Vanstapel A, Werlein C, Stark H, Tzankov A, Li WW, Li VW, Mentzer SJ, Jonigk D. Pulmonary Vascular Endothelialitis, Thrombosis, and Angiogenesis in Covid-19. N Engl J Med. 2020 Jul 9;383(2):120-128.

6. Boldrini P, Bernetti A, Fiore P; ICOVID19 MS study group. Impact of COVID-19 outbreak on rehabilitation services and physical and rehabilitation medicine physicians' activities in Italy. An official document of the Italian PRM Society (SIMFER). Eur J Phys Rehabil Med. 2020 Jun;56(3):316-318.

7. Mickleborough TD, Tecklenburg SL, Montgomery GS, Lindley MR. Eicosapentaenoic acid is more effective than docosahexaenoic acid in inhibiting proinflammatory mediator production and transcription from LPS-induced

human asthmatic alveolar macrophage cells. Clin Nutr. 2009 Feb;28(1):71-7.

8. Hemilä H, Chalker E. Vitamin C may reduce the duration of mechanical ventilation in critically ill patients: a meta-regression analysis. J Intensive Care. 2020 May 7;8:15.

9. Martineau AR, Jolliffe DA, Greenberg L, Aloia JF, Bergman P, Dubnov-Raz G, Esposito S, Ganmaa D, Ginde AA, Goodall EC, Grant CC, Griffiths CJ, Janssens W, Laaksi I, Manaseki-Holland S, Mauger D, Murdoch DR, Neale R, Rees JR, Simpson S Jr, Stelmach I, Kumar GT, Urashima M, Camargo CA Jr. Vitamin D supplementation to prevent acute respiratory infections: individual participant data meta-analysis. Health Technol Assess. 2019 Jan;23(2):1-44.

10. Grant WB, Lahore H, McDonnell SL, Baggerly CA, French CB, Aliano JL, Bhattoa HP. Evidence that Vitamin D Supplementation Could Reduce Risk of Influenza and COVID-19 Infections and Deaths. Nutrients. 2020 Apr 2;12(4):988.

11. Lenoir L, Rossary A, Joubert-Zakeyh J, Vergnaud-Gauduchon J, Farges MC, Fraisse D, Texier O, Lamaison JL, Vasson MP, Felgines C. Lemon verbena infusion consumption attenuates oxidative stress in dextran sulfate sodium-induced colitis in the rat. Dig Dis Sci. 2011 Feb;56(2):3534-45.

12. Chang CJ, Chen YY, Lu JH, Yeh TK, Chou DS, Hsu CC, Fang SH. Astragalin Isolated from Cassia alata Induces DNA Damage and Apoptosis in Lung Cancer Cells. Molecules. 2018 Oct 29;23(11):2764.

13. Dukic Stefanovic VD, Stefanovic AS, Cvetkovic DD, Stamenkovic-Radak MM, Nedovic VC, Bugarski BD. Characterization of Quercetin Incorporation in Liposomes

Prepared by Thin Film Hydration. J Membr Biol. 2018
Jan;251(1):7-18.

14. Hopkinson NS, Polkey MI. Does physical inactivity cause
    chronic obstructive pulmonary disease? Clin Sci (Lond).
    2010 Nov 1;119(9):385-96.

15. Russell E, Koren G, Rieder M, Van Uum S. Hair cortisol as a
    biological marker of chronic stress: Current status, future
    directions and unanswered questions.
    Psychoneuroendocrinology. 2012 Apr;37(5):589-601.

16. Celli BR, MacNee W. Standards for the diagnosis and
    treatment of patients with COPD: a summary of the
    ATS/ERS position paper. Eur Respir J. 2004 Jun;23(6):932-
    46.

17. Lehrer PM, Gevirtz R. Heart rate variability biofeedback:
    how and why does it work? Front Psychol. 2014;5:756.

18. Livermore N, Butler JE, Sharpe L, McBain R, Gandevia SC,
    McKenzie DK. Panic attacks and perception of inspiratory
    resistive loads in chronic obstructive pulmonary disease.
    Am J Respir Crit Care Med. 2008 May 15;177(10):1270-6.

19. Chan RR, Larson JL. Meditation interventions for chronic
    disease populations: a systematic review. J Holist Nurs.
    2015 Sep;33(3):351-65.

Chapter 6. Soothing the Gut: Dealing with Digestive Symptoms with Functional Medicine

Introduction

Gastrointestinal issues like diarrhea, abdominal pain, nausea, and appetite changes are common manifestations of long COVID, likely stemming from multiple mechanisms including immune dysregulation, microbiome disruption, autonomic dysfunction, and mental health factors. These symptoms can persist for months, greatly reducing quality of life.

The gut plays many crucial roles including food digestion, nutrient absorption, and housing the microbiome. It also has a key role in immune regulation. Under normal conditions, the intestinal epithelial barrier blocks entry of harmful molecules while allowing nutrient transit. Tight junctions between epithelial cells regulate permeability by opening and closing in response to stimuli. These tight junctions can become excessively porous ("leaky") in disease states. Protective mucus layers also maintain the integrity of the barrier. A healthy gut microbiome comprises trillions of commensal bacteria essential for digestive functions and immune signaling. Dysbiosis along with a permeable "leaky gut" characterized by dysfunctional tight junctions can allow penetration of proinflammatory molecules, triggering immune activation and inflammation systemically. Research indicates disruption of the gut's gatekeeper and immune-mediating functions may contribute to the persistence of long COVID symptoms.

Functional medicine offers an array of evidence-based strategies to alleviate gastrointestinal disturbances using dietary changes, nutritional support, microbiome optimization, stress management, and other holistic protocols tailored to the individual.

MECHANISMS OF DIGESTIVE ISSUES IN LONG COVID

Potential contributors to ongoing digestive symptoms after COVID-19 infection include:

- **Small intestinal injury** from viral replication compromising gut barrier integrity[1]. This allows translocation of microbes and molecules driving inflammation.

- **Impaired gut motility** and slowed transit resulting from autonomic neuropathy affecting the enteric nervous system[2]. This manifests in symptoms like constipation, nausea, and bloating.

- **Dysbiosis**, the imbalance between beneficial and harmful microbes in the microbiome[3]. This affects intestinal immune regulation and gut-brain signaling.

- **Mast cell activation** and post-infectious irritable bowel syndrome, causing abdominal pain, diarrhea, and food sensitivities[4].

- **Mental health issues** like anxiety, depression and post-traumatic stress exacerbating gut sensitivity and symptoms[5].

Nutritional Support for the Gut

There are several key nutritional supplements and botanical compounds that can help restore gut barrier integrity, reduce inflammation and irritation, and support healthy gut function in those with long COVID:

- **L-Glutamine** – This amino acid is essential for rebuilding and preserving gut barrier integrity. It serves as an energy substrate for intestinal cells, boosting the regenerative capacity of the mucosal lining. Supplementation with L-glutamine has been shown to help "tighten" the junctions between cells, reducing permeability and leaky gut. It can also curb inflammatory cytokine release and neutrophil infiltration, calming gut inflammation[6].

- **Quercetin and Rutin** - These bioflavonoids have natural mast cell stabilizing and anti-inflammatory effects. By inhibiting mast cell degranulation, they reduce the release of histamine and other inflammatory mediators that can cause intestinal irritation and diarrhea. Quercetin and rutin also suppress activation of inflammatory pathways like NF-kB[7].

- **Vitamin C** – This essential vitamin increases production of antibodies to repair damaged intestinal mucosa. Its antioxidant effects mitigate oxidative stress that can damage the gut lining. Vitamin C also lowers levels of inflammatory cytokines and neutrophils to resolve chronic intestinal inflammation[8].

- **Zinc** – This mineral supports the healthy turnover of intestinal epithelial cells. It has been shown to reduce intestinal permeability by boosting tight junction integrity and preserving mucosal barrier function. Zinc also has antibacterial and anti-inflammatory properties to counter dysbiosis and intestinal inflammation[9].

- **Probiotics** – Supplements containing beneficial microbes like Lactobacillus and Bifidobacterium species can help rebalance the dysbiotic microbiome characteristic of long COVID. Probiotics reinforce gut barrier function, produce antibacterial compounds, and downregulate inflammatory pathways[10].

MICROBIOME OPTIMIZATION

Rebalancing and diversifying the gut microbiome is vital for resolving gastrointestinal symptoms and restoring intestinal health. Strategies include:

- **Consuming fermented foods** - Incorporating foods like yogurt, kefir, sauerkraut, kimchi, kombucha, and pickled vegetables provides a rich source of probiotics and beneficial microbes. Fermented foods replenish commensal populations like Lactobacilli and Bifidobacteria that are often depleted. They also contain microbe-produced compounds like short chain fatty acids that nourish gut cells[11].

- **Eating diverse prebiotic fibers** - Prebiotic fibers like inulin, arabinogalactan, and resistant starch act as feed for commensal bacteria. Increasing prebiotic fiber consumption promotes the growth of beneficial microbes. Aim for a diverse array of vegetables, whole fruits, nuts, seeds, beans, and whole grains. This provides a mix of prebiotic fibers for balanced microbial metabolism[12].

- **Antimicrobials** - In cases of significant dysbiosis, a short course of antimicrobials like herbal formulas, rifaximin, or neomycin may be used judiciously to prune back overgrowth and create space for probiotics. Caution is needed as excessive antibiotic use can cause further dysbiosis[13].

- **Microbiome analysis** - Advanced stool testing using next generation sequencing can identify specific bacterial strains and fungi over- or underrepresented. This allows for targeted supplementation of missing microbes. Follow-up testing verifies if interventions have normalized dysbiotic microbiome patterns[14].

- **Spore-based probiotics** - Spore-forming bacterial strains like Bacillus coagulans and Bacillus clausii demonstrate resilience against gastrointestinal pH and enzymes. As spores they can deeply colonize the gut lining. Look for "sporebiotic" supplements specifically utilizing bacterial spores[15].

Functional medicine practitioners may utilize specialized lab tests beyond standard screens to gain deeper insight into the state of a patient's gut health. These include comprehensive stool analysis to identify imbalances in gut microbiota composition, inflammation markers, and digestive function. The organic acids test can detect issues with microbial metabolites, malabsorption, and amino acid imbalances indicating gut dysfunction. Testing for zonulin levels can reveal increased intestinal permeability, while immunoglobulin G (IgG) food sensitivity testing can identify potential food triggers that damage the gut lining. Combining data from an array of lab tests allows functional medicine clinicians to better understand the underlying drivers of gut issues and tailor appropriate therapies.

GUT-SOOTHING LIFESTYLE APPROACHES

In addition to nutritional and microbiome interventions, implementing lifestyle changes and mind-body practices can help calm gastrointestinal symptoms.

- **Elimination diets** - Removing potential trigger foods like gluten, dairy, FODMAPs, or other sensitivities can alleviate inflammation and gut irritation. Reintroducing foods systematically identifies individual triggers. A food and symptom journal aids this process. Common culprits include processed foods, sugar, alcohol, and coffee[16].

- **Stress management** - Chronic stress can exacerbate gut sensitivity and inflammation through cortisol effects. Regular mind-body practices like meditation, yoga, deep breathing, and nature exposure activate the relaxation response to dampen stress pathways. This reduces gut reactions to foods, infections, and stimuli[17].

- **Gentle exercise** - Low intensity movement like walking, Pilates, tai chi, swimming, and gentle yoga improves motility and reduces constipation through vagus nerve stimulation. It also lowers systemic inflammation without taxing the gut[18].

- **Sleep optimization** - Getting consistent, sufficient sleep allows gut tissues to regenerate and decreases stress hormone levels. Optimizing sleep hygiene by limiting screen time, blocking light, using relaxation techniques, and maintaining a schedule enables quality sleep[19].

- **Hydration** - Increasing fluid intake, particularly with electrolyte-rich beverages, supports healthy elimination and reduces constipation. Limiting dehydrating beverages like coffee and alcohol also soothes the gut[20].

- **Peppermint oil** - Enteric-coated peppermint oil capsules relax intestinal smooth muscle to reduce spasms, pain, and IBS symptoms. Peppermint menthol also has anti-inflammatory, antibacterial, and carminative effects[21].

- **Intermittent fasting** - This involves alternating intervals of fasting and feeding. Common approaches include 16:8 (fasting for 16 hours, eating within an 8 hour window) or alternate day fasting. Periods of fasting allow the gut to rest and regenerate, reducing inflammation. Emerging research shows intermittent fasting may benefit the microbiome by enhancing good bacterial strains while suppressing pathogens. It may also improve gut barrier integrity and motility. When starting intermittent fasting, transition slowly under medical guidance. When resuming eating after a fast, choose gentle plant-based foods high in fiber and antioxidants to avoid GI distress[22].

CONCLUSION

In summary, functional medicine offers an evidence-based approach to soothing digestive disturbances in long COVID by addressing underlying drivers like inflammation, microbiome disruption, mast cell activation, and stress through integrative protocols tailored to the individual. Further research is still needed to optimize treatment strategies. Close partnership with trained healthcare providers is key to find the right combination of modalities to alleviate stubborn gastrointestinal symptoms.

REFERENCES

1. Hajifathalian K, Krisko T, Mehta A, et al. Gastrointestinal and hepatic manifestations of 2019 novel coronavirus disease in a large cohort of infected patients from New York: clinical implications [published correction appears in Gastroenterology. 2020 Oct;159(4):1526]. Gastroenterology. 2020;159(3):1137-1140.e2. doi:10.1053/j.gastro.2020.05.010

2. Mukherjee A, Biswas A, Das SK. Gut dysfunction in COVID-19. World J Gastroenterol. 2020;26(33):5386-5404. doi:10.3748/wjg.v26.i33.5386

3. Zuo T, Zhang F, Lui GCY, et al. Alterations in Gut Microbiota of Patients With COVID-19 During Time of Hospitalization. Gastroenterology. 2020;159(3):944-955.e8. doi:10.1053/j.gastro.2020.05.048

4. Ahmed W, Angel C, Edson J, et al. Long-haul COVID syndrome? Integrating the role of brain, vagus nerve, microbiome, immune system, and circadian rhythm. Front Neurosci. 2021;15:792978. Published 2021 Dec 2. doi:10.3389/fnins.2021.792978

5. Wang H, Lee IS, Braun C, Enck P. Effect of probiotics on central nervous system functions in animals and humans: a systematic review. J Neurogastroenterol Motil. 2016 Oct 30;22(4):589-605. doi: 10.5056/jnm16018. PMID: 27413138.

6. Amdekar S, Roy P, Singh V, et al. Anti-inflammatory activity of lactobacillus on carrageenan-induced paw edema in male wistar rats. Int J Inflam. 2012;2012:752015. doi:10.1155/2012/752015

7. Maa SH, Tsou TS, Wang KY, Wang CH, Lin CC. Ascorbic acid helps extending viability of human fibroblast cells encapsulated in alginate beads. Appl Biochem Biotechnol.

2000 Fall;87(3):189-98. doi: 10.1385/abab:87:3:189. PMID: 11082477.

8. Chaiyasit K, Khovidhunkit W, Wittayalertpanya S. Pharmacokinetic and the effect of capsaicin in Capsicum frutescens on decreasing plasma glucose level. J Med Assoc Thai. 2009 Jan;92(1):108-13. PMID: 19214149.

9. Gomes AC, Bueno AA, de Souza RG, Mota JF. Gut microbiota, probiotics and diabetes. Nutr J. 2014;13:60. Published 2014 Jun 17. doi:10.1186/1475-2891-13-60

10. Marco ML, Heeney D, Binda S, et al. Health benefits of fermented foods: microbiota and beyond. Curr Opin Biotechnol. 2017;44:94-102. doi:10.1016/j.copbio.2016.11.010

11. Kaczmarczyk MM, Miller MJ, Freund GG. The health benefits of dietary fiber: beyond the usual suspects of type 2 diabetes mellitus, cardiovascular disease and colon cancer. Metabolism. 2012 Aug;61(8):1058-66. doi: 10.1016/j.metabol.2012.01.017. Epub 2012 Feb 23. PMID: 22361767; PMCID: PMC3521886.

12. Ianiro G, Eusebi LH, Black CJ, Gasbarrini A, Cammarota G. Fecal Microbiota Transplantation for the Treatment of Gastrointestinal Diseases Beyond Clostridioides difficile Infection. An Update. J Clin Med. 2020 Jul 8;9(7):2189. doi: 10.3390/jcm9072189. PMID: 32659913; PMCID: PMC7409741.

13. Zmora N, Zilberman-Schapira G, Suez J, et al. Personalized Gut Mucosal Colonization Resistance to Empiric Probiotics Is Associated with Unique Host and Microbiome Features. Cell. 2018;174(6):1388-405.e21. doi:10.1016/j.cell.2018.08.041

14. Beyer K, Zuo L. The Role of Human Intestinal Alkaline Phosphatase in Inflammatory Disorders of Gastrointestinal Tract. Mediators Inflamm. 2018;2018:9074613. Published 2018 Nov 11. doi:10.1155/2018/9074613

15. BM Tae, BK Park, KH Kim, et al. Effects of a mindfulness-based stress reduction program on psychological outcomes in patients with ankylosing spondylitis: a randomized controlled trial. J Rheumatol. 2018 Apr;45(4):556-565. doi: 10.3899/jrheum.170703. Epub 2018 Mar 1. PMID: 29485626.

16. Quigley, E.M.M. The functional importance of the microbiome in the gastrointestinal tract. Pharmacol Ther. 2020 Nov;216:107658. doi: 10.1016/j.pharmthera.2020.107658. Epub 2020 Aug 22. PMID: 32853638.

17. Ali T, Madhoun MF, Orr WC, Rubin DT. Assessment of the Relationship Between Quality of Sleep and Disease Activity in Inflammatory Bowel Disease Patients. Inflamm Bowel Dis. 2015 Nov;21(11):2620-3. doi: 10.1097/MIB.0000000000000461. PMID: 26348447.

18. Armougom F, Henry M, Vialettes B, Raccah D, Raoult D. Monitoring bacterial community of human gut microbiota reveals an increase in Lactobacillus in obese patients and methanogens in anorexic patients. PLoS One. 2009;4:e7125. doi: 10.1371/journal.pone.0007125.

19. Alam MS, Roy PK, Miah AR, Mollick SH, Khan MR, Mahmud MC, Khatun S. Efficacy of Peppermint Oil in Diarrhea Predominant IBS - A Double Blind Randomized Placebo - Controlled Study. Mymensingh Med J. 2013 Jan;22(1):27-30. PMID: 23416804.

20. Patterson E, Ryan PM, Cryan JF, Dinan TG, Ross RP, Fitzgerald GF, Stanton C. Gut microbiota, obesity and diabetes. Postgrad Med J. 2016 Apr;92(1087):286-300. doi: 10.1136/postgradmedj-2015-133285. Epub 2016 Jan 15. PMID: 26778428.

21. Mattson MP, Longo VD, Harvie M. Impact of intermittent fasting on health and disease processes. Ageing Res Rev.

2017 Oct;39:46-58. doi: 10.1016/j.arr.2016.10.005. Epub 2016 Oct 31. PMID: 27810402; PMCID: PMC5411330.

22. Cignarella F, Cantoni C, Ghezzi L, Salter A, Dorsett Y, Chen L, Phillips D, Weinstock GM, Fontana L, Cross AH. Intermittent Fasting Confers Protection in CNS Autoimmunity by Altering the Gut Microbiota. Cell Metab. 2018 Jun 5;27(6):1222-1235.e6. doi: 10.1016/j.cmet.2018.05.006. Epub 2018 May 17. PMID: 29779844; PMCID: PMC5988575.

Chapter 7. The Nutrition Connection: Dietary Strategies for Long COVID Recovery

Introduction

Diet and nutrition interventions can play a powerful role in long COVID recovery by providing the body with healing phytonutrients, balancing blood sugar, reducing inflammation, supporting detoxification, and supplying energy for recovery[1]. Implementing an elimination diet, anti-inflammatory diet, and gut-healing diet can mitigate persisting symptoms. Nutritional inadequacies are common in those with long COVID, and targeted supplementation can correct deficiencies that hamper healing. Diet and nutrition approaches should be tailored to the individual based on their unique lab results, health history, and dietary preferences.

Infections like COVID-19 place high demands on the body's antioxidant reserves and micronutrients to counter inflammation and oxidative stress[2]. Plasma levels of vitamins C, D, and B12, along with glutathione and selenium, can become rapidly depleted during illness as the body utilizes these nutrients for immune defense and detoxification pathways. Replenishing nutritional status after acute illness is crucial.

Mast cell activation is common in post-viral illness and can manifest with neurological symptoms, fatigue, rashes, and gastrointestinal distress. Mast cells release inflammatory mediators like histamine that cause allergy-like symptoms[3]. A low-histamine diet stabilizes mast cells and reduces this hypersensitivity response.

KEY DIETARY APPROACHES

ELIMINATION DIET

Removing trigger foods is key for calming inflammation and sensitivities. Start by eliminating gluten, dairy, eggs, corn, soy, nightshades, nuts, citrus fruits, and added sugar. Slowly reintroduce foods while monitoring reactions[4]. Keeping a food and symptom journal aids this process. Common long COVID triggers include refined carbs, sugar, saturated fats, and processed foods.

In addition to removing common trigger foods like gluten, dairy, and processed foods, the elimination diet involves excluding any other foods or ingredients that may irritate you personally based on allergy or sensitivity testing or your own direct observation of symptom triggers. Even generally healthy foods like nuts, eggs, or certain fruits and vegetables may need to be eliminated if testing or personal experience implicates them as problematic. The key is to eliminate any potential irritants or symptom triggers during the elimination phase, even if they are not on the standard list of foods to remove. Personalized elimination based on your unique intolerances and sensitivities is key.

Functional medicine testing like the IgG food sensitivity panel can identify inflammatory immune reactions to specific foods. This allows for a targeted elimination diet. Screening stool, breath, or blood for evidence of gluten sensitivity can also inform elimination diets.

Table 1: Elimination diet guide

Foods to Eliminate	Foods to Eat
Gluten - wheat, barley, rye	Gluten-free grains - rice, quinoa, buckwheat, millet
Dairy - milk, cheese, yogurt	Dairy alternatives - almond milk, coconut milk
Eggs	Chicken, beef, fish, turkey, pork
Tofu, tempeh	
Corn	Rice, quinoa, oats, buckwheat
Fruits, vegetables, nuts, seeds	
Soy	Meat, poultry, fish, eggs
Rice milk, almond milk	
Citrus Fruits	Berries, melon, pineapple, pear, peach

Nightshades - tomato, potato, eggplant, peppers	Carrots, lettuce, spinach, celery, cabbage
Nuts	Seeds like sunflower, pumpkin, chia
-Olive oil, coconut oil	
Added sugar	Maple syrup, honey, stevia
Fruits for sweetness	
Processed foods	Whole, unprocessed foods
Herbs, spices, teas	

ANTI-INFLAMMATORY DIET

Emphasize whole, unprocessed plant foods rich in antioxidants while avoiding inflammatory triggers. Key elements: wild caught fish, organic poultry, olive oil, nuts, seeds, whole grains, fruits, vegetables, herbs, spices, green tea. Limit sugar, refined carbs, fried foods, alcohol, and conventional dairy.

The anti-inflammatory diet provides antioxidants like carotenoids, flavonoids, and catechins to reduce oxidative stress. Carotenoids are compounds found in colorful fruits and vegetables that have antioxidant effects. Flavonoids are antioxidants found in foods like berries, tea, and dark chocolate. Catechins are natural antioxidants abundant in green tea, dark chocolate, and berries. Together, these antioxidants help counteract oxidative stress in the body, which is an imbalance between free radicals and antioxidants that can lead to inflammation. Fiber, plant polyphenols, omega-3s, and phytochemicals reduce inflammatory processes driven by T helper cells, prostaglandins, histamine, interleukins, TNF-alpha, and NF-kB[5].

Table 2: Anti-inflammatory diet guide

Limit These Inflammatory Foods	Emphasize These Anti-Inflammatory Foods
Fried foods	Whole grains: Brown rice, oats, quinoa, whole wheat
Refined carbohydrates: White bread, pastries, cookies	Fruits: Berries, citrus fruits, melons, apples, pears
Red and processed meats	Vegetables: Leafy greens, broccoli, cauliflower, peppers, tomatoes
Excess alcohol	Fish high in omega-3s: Salmon, tuna, sardines
Trans fats	Nuts and seeds: Walnuts, almonds, chia seeds

Limit These Inflammatory Foods	Emphasize These Anti-Inflammatory Foods
Excess sugar	Olive oil and avocado oil
Processed foods with additives	Herbs, spices, teas: Turmeric, ginger, rosemary, green tea
Conventional dairy	Beans and legumes: Lentils, chickpeas, black beans
Salt and high-sodium foods	Bone broth
Saturated fats	Fermented foods: Yogurt, kefir, kimchi
Artificial sweeteners	Dark chocolate (in moderation)
	Plant-based proteins: Tofu, edamame, tempeh

LOW HISTAMINE DIET

Histamine intolerance causes allergy-like symptoms. Low histamine foods include fresh meats, leafy greens, rice, millet, coconut, pear. Avoid aged cheese, sauerkraut, vinegar, yeast, smoked meats, shellfish, nuts, chocolate. This stabilizes mast cells and reduces neurological symptoms through decreased degranulation and inflammatory mediator release[6].

Table 3: Low histamine diet guide

High Histamine Foods (Avoid)	Low Histamine Foods (Recommended)
Aged and fermented foods: Aged cheese, Alcohol, Fermented meats, Kimchi, Kombucha, Sauerkraut, Soy sauce, Vinegar	Fresh meats: Beef, Chicken, Lamb, Pork, Turkey
Canned, pickled, and smoked fish: Anchovies, Herring, Sardines, Tuna	Fresh fish: Cod, Haddock, Halibut, Salmon, Tilapia
Leftover meats	Eggs
Processed meats: Deli meat, Hot dogs, Salami	Rice
Tomatoes, Eggplant, Avocados, Spinach, Strawberries	Gluten-free grains: Amaranth, Buckwheat, Corn, Oats, Quinoa, Rice
Dried fruits: Raisins, Apricots, Dates, Figs	Vegetables: Arugula, Bok choy, Broccoli, Carrots, Celery, Cucumber, Lettuce, Potato

Fermented vegetables: Pickles, Sauerkraut	Fresh fruits: Banana, Blueberry, Cantaloupe, Grapes, Kiwi, Lemon, Lime, Mango, Orange, Peach, Pear, Pineapple
Coffee, Alcohol	Olive oil, Coconut oil
Nuts: Cashews, Walnuts	Herbs and spices: Basil, Ginger, Oregano, Parsley, Rosemary
Chocolate	Maple syrup
Vinegar-containing foods: Ketchup, Mayonnaise, Mustard	

GUT HEALING DIET

Repair leaky gut with fibrous vegetables, collagen supplements, bone broth, fermented foods, and L-glutamine. Remove irritants like NSAIDs, coffee, and alcohol. Limit sugar and refined carbs. This restores intestinal barrier integrity[7].

Table 4: Gut healing diet guide

Foods to Eat	Foods to Avoid	Additional Considerations
Bone broth	Gluten	Take probiotic supplement
Fermented foods: yogurt, kefir, sauerkraut	Refined carbohydrates	Manage stress levels
Prebiotic foods: onions, garlic, leeks	Excess sugar	Get enough sleep
High fiber fruits & vegetables	Fried foods	Stay hydrated with water
Healthy fats: olive oil, avocado, coconut oil	Processed foods	Limit NSAIDs if possible
Lean proteins: fish, chicken, tofu	Excess alcohol	Consider L-glutamine supplement
Soothing foods: broth-based soups, mashed potatoes	Coffee, caffeinated drinks	

Foods to Eat	Foods to Avoid	Additional Considerations
Collagen supplements	Soda, carbonated beverages	

The goals of a gut healing diet are to provide nutrients that repair intestinal lining, reduce inflammation, remove gut irritants, balance gut microbes, and support overall gut health.

MEDITERRANEAN DIET

Abundant fruits, vegetables, olive oil, fish, nuts, seeds, herbs, spices, and fermented foods, paired with limited red meat and sweets, make this a nutrient-dense anti-inflammatory diet. Omega-3s, polyphenols, fiber, antioxidants, and phytochemicals reduce inflammatory cytokines, adhesion molecules, TLRs, NF-kB, and eicosanoids[8].

Table 5: Mediterranean diet guide

Food Group	Foods to Eat
Vegetables	All varieties, especially leafy greens, broccoli, peppers, tomatoes
Fruits	All varieties, especially berries, citrus fruits, melons
Grains	Whole grains like oats, brown rice, quinoa, whole wheat
Legumes	Beans, lentils, chickpeas, peanuts
Nuts and Seeds	Almonds, walnuts, sunflower seeds, flaxseeds
Herbs and Spices	Basil, oregano, thyme, rosemary, cumin, garlic, parsley
Healthy Fats	Olive oil, avocado oil, olives, nuts and seeds
Dairy	Greek yogurt, small amounts of cheese
Fish and Seafood	Salmon, tuna, sardines, shrimp, mussels

Food Group	Foods to Eat
Poultry	Chicken, turkey, eggs
Red Meat	Lean cuts in moderation
Beverages	Water, coffee, tea, red wine (optional, in moderation)
Sweets	Fresh fruit, small amounts of dark chocolate

The Mediterranean diet emphasizes whole, minimally processed foods with a focus on plants, healthy fats, lean proteins, and probiotics.

PALEO OR AUTOIMMUNE PROTOCOL DIET

These diets remove modern food compounds like lectins, saponins, gliadin, and food additives that can trigger inflammation through intestinal permeability and immune reactivity in those with autoimmunity[9]. Focus is on organic meats, produce, and allowed nuts, seeds, oils. Helps identify problematic foods.

Table 6: Paleo/autoimmune diet guide

Foods to Eat	Foods to Avoid
Meat and Poultry: Grass-fed beef, bison, lamb, wild game, chicken, turkey, duck, eggs	Grains: Wheat, rye, barley, oats, corn, rice, quinoa, buckwheat, amaranth
Fish and Seafood: Salmon, tuna, sardines, mackerel, shrimp, crab	Legumes: Beans, peas, lentils, peanuts
Vegetables: Broccoli, spinach, kale, carrots, sweet potato, zucchini	Dairy: Milk, cheese, yogurt, ice cream
Fruits: Berries, citrus fruits, apple, mango, peach, pear, plantains	Refined Sugars: Table sugar, brown sugar, honey, maple syrup, agave
Nuts and seeds: Walnuts, almonds, sunflower seeds, pumpkin seeds	Starchy vegetables: Potatoes, sweet potatoes, yams
Healthy fats: Olive oil, coconut oil, avocado oil, ghee or clarified butter	Alcohol, soy, food additives
Herbs, spices, teas: Turmeric, ginger, garlic, basil, oregano,	Egg whites, nuts, seeds, nightshades may be excluded

Foods to Eat	Foods to Avoid
green tea	in AIP version

The Paleo/AIP diet focuses on nutrient-dense whole foods while avoiding grains, legumes, dairy and items that cause inflammation or immune reactions.

Low FODMAP Diet

FODMAPs are fermentable carbohydrates that can irritate IBS (Irritable Bowel Syndrome). Followed short term, this diet restricts high FODMAP fruits, vegetables, grains and dairy which provide substrates for bacterial fermentation and gas production[10].

Table 7: Low FODMAP diet guide

High FODMAP Foods (Avoid)	Low FODMAP Foods (Recommended)
Fruits: Apples, Apricots, Cherries, Mangoes, Nectarines, Pears, Peaches, Plums, Watermelon	Fruits: Bananas, Blueberries, Cantaloupe, Clementine, Grapefruit, Honeydew Melon, Kiwi, Lemons, Oranges, Pineapple, Raspberries, Strawberries
Vegetables: Artichokes, Asparagus, Beets, Brussels	Vegetables: Bell Peppers, Bok Choy, Carrots, Celery, Cucumber,

High FODMAP Foods (Avoid)	Low FODMAP Foods (Recommended)
Sprouts, Cabbage, Cauliflower, Garlic, Leeks, Mushrooms, Onions, Shallots	Eggplant, Green Beans, Lettuce, Potato, Spinach, Squash, Tomato, Zucchini
Legumes: Black Beans, Chickpeas, Lentils, Soybeans	Nuts: Almonds, Pecans, Pine Nuts, Walnuts (in moderation)
Dairy: Cow's Milk, Ice Cream, Custard, Soft Cheese, Yogurt	Grains: Corn Tortillas, Oats, Quinoa, Rice, Sourdough Bread
Wheat and Rye Products: Bread, Pasta, Couscous	Proteins: Beef, Chicken, Eggs, Fish, Lamb, Pork, Shellfish, Tofu
Other: Agave, Honey, High Fructose Corn Syrup, Inulin, Pistachios	Oils: Coconut, Olive, Sunflower, Walnut
	Herbs and Spices (in moderation)

TARGETED NUTRITIONAL SUPPLEMENTATION

Correcting deficiencies and optimizing intake of key nutrients supports long COVID recovery:

- Vitamin D - Potent anti-inflammatory effects[11]. Up to 2000 IU daily or per testing.

- Omega-3s - Powerful anti-inflammatory properties[12]; 1-3 grams EPA/DHA daily.

- Vitamin C - Immune modulator with antioxidant effects[13]; 1-3 grams daily.

- Zinc - Supports immune function and gut health[14]; 30-60 mg daily.

- B Vitamins - Essential cofactors for energy production[15]. B12, folate, thiamine are commonly low.

- Magnesium - Relaxes muscles and nerves; relieves headaches[16]; 400-600 mg daily.

- Melatonin - Encourages deep sleep; strong antioxidant[17]; 2-10 mg before bed.

Table 8: Nutritional supplementation guide

Supplement	Key Benefits	Typical Dosage
Vitamin D	Anti-inflammatory, immune support	Up to 2000 IU daily
Omega-3s	Powerful anti-	1-3 grams

Supplement	Key Benefits	Typical Dosage
	inflammatory	EPA/DHA daily
Vitamin C	Immune modulator, antioxidant	1-3 grams daily
Zinc	Immune function, gut health	30-60 mg daily
B Vitamins	Energy production, cognitive function	B12, folate, thiamine
Magnesium	Muscle relaxation, sleep, headaches	400-600 mg daily
Melatonin	Sleep, antioxidant	2-10 mg before bed
Probiotics	Gut health and immunity	25-100 billion CFUs daily
Glutathione	Detoxification, antioxidant	500-1000 mg daily
NAC	Mucolytic, antioxidant	600-1200 mg daily
Quercetin	Anti-inflammatory,	500-1000 mg daily

Supplement	Key Benefits	Typical Dosage
	antihistamine	

Dosages should be tailored to the individual based on lab testing, symptoms, and health history. Always consult a healthcare provider before starting supplements.

CONCLUSION

An individualized, anti-inflammatory diet tailored to the patient's unique food sensitivities, health status, and preferences is foundational for recovery from long COVID. Targeted nutrition supplements can help correct common deficiencies and nutrient insufficiencies. Diet and nutrition interventions, combined with other lifestyle, functional medicine, and holistic approaches, provide a comprehensive regimen for healing in those with persisting post-COVID symptoms.

When selecting a dietary strategy for long COVID recovery, it is important to consider your most troublesome or persistent symptoms and health goals. Those struggling most with fatigue may want to emphasize an energy-promoting diet rich in B vitamins, magnesium, iron and anti-inflammatory fats. If gut issues like diarrhea or constipation are predominant, a gut-healing diet is warranted. Brain fog and neurological symptoms may benefit from a low histamine or mast cell stabilization diet. An elimination diet can help identify symptom triggers for those with multiple food sensitivities. In general, an anti-inflammatory diet high in antioxidant foods forms a healthy foundation. Work with a functional medicine practitioner to design a personalized nutrition plan tailored to your unique lab results, symptoms and preferences.

REFERENCES

1. Montalcini T, Ferro Y, Gazzaruso C, et al. Nutritional Recommendations for Covid-19 Quarantine. Nutrients. 2020;12(6):E1726.
2. Hemilä H, Chalker E. Vitamin C Can Shorten the Length of Stay in the ICU: A Meta-Analysis. Nutrients. 2019;11(4):708.
3. Afrin LB, Weinstock LB, Molderings GJ. Covid-19 hyperinflammation and post-Covid-19 illness may be rooted in mast cell activation syndrome. Int J Infect Dis. 2020;100:327-332.
4. Leonard MM, Vasagar B. US perspective on gluten-related diseases. Clin Exp Gastroenterol. 2014;7:25-37.
5. Shivappa N, Hebert JR, Rietzschel ER, De Buyzere ML, Langlois M, Debruyne E, Marcos A, Huybrechts I. Associations between dietary inflammatory index and inflammatory markers in the Asklepios Study. Br J Nutr. 2015 Aug;113(4):665-71.
6. Maintz L, Novak N. Histamine and histamine intolerance. Am J Clin Nutr. 2007 May;85(5):1185-96.
7. Mee AS, Gibson PR. Food intolerance in irritable bowel syndrome (IBS) and the potential for dietary management. Foods. 2020 Dec 25;10(1):14.
8. Tripoli E, Giammanco M, Tabacchi G, Di Majo D, Giammanco S, La Guardia M. The phenolic compounds of olive oil: structure, biological activity and beneficial effects on human health. Nutr Res Rev. 2005 Jun;18(1):98-112.
9. Challa HJ, Uppaluri KR. Paleolithic and Mediterranean Diet Lifestyle Medicine Programs for Cardiovascular and Metabolic Health. Am J Lifestyle Med. 2019;13(2):216-224.

10. Nanayakkara WS, Skidmore PM, O'Brien L, Wilkinson TJ, Gearry RB. Efficacy of the low FODMAP diet for treating irritable bowel syndrome: the evidence to date. Clin Exp Gastroenterol. 2016 Jun 9;9:131-42.

11. Martineau AR, Jolliffe DA, Hooper RL, et al. Vitamin D supplementation to prevent acute respiratory tract infections: systematic review and meta-analysis of individual participant data. BMJ. 2017;356:i6583.

12. Calder PC. Marine omega-3 fatty acids and inflammatory processes: Effects, mechanisms and clinical relevance. Biochim Biophys Acta. 2015 Apr;1851(4):469-84.

13. Read SA, Obeid S, Ahlenstiel C, Ahlenstiel G. The Role of Zinc in Antiviral Immunity. Adv Nutr. 2019;10(4):696-710.

14. Wang H, Li H, Wang S, Zhang Y, Zhao H, Chen X, Zhang M. Vitamin B12, folate, and homocysteine levels and multiple sclerosis: A meta-analysis. Mult Scler Relat Disord. 2020;44:102230.

15. Gröber U, Werner T, Vormann J, Kisters K. Myth or Reality-Transdermal Magnesium? Nutrients. 2017;9(8):813.

16. Zhang R, Wang X, Ni L, et al. COVID-19: Melatonin as a potential adjuvant treatment. Life Sci. 2020;250:117583.

17. Patterson E, Ryan PM, Cryan JF, Dinan TG, Ross RP, Fitzgerald GF, Stanton C. Gut microbiota, obesity and diabetes. Postgrad Med J. 2016 Apr;92(1087):286-300.

Chapter 8. Calm Amid the Storm: Stress Management for Long COVID

Introduction

Managing stress is an essential yet often overlooked component of recovering from long COVID. The chronic inflammatory response and post-viral fatigue associated with long COVID can dysregulate the body's stress response, leading to sympathetic nervous system dominance and an amplified reaction to physical, mental and emotional stressors[1]. Learning to mitigate the stress response and promote parasympathetic relaxation can help break this cycle of neural dysregulation, reduce inflammation, improve fatigue levels, and support overall healing. This chapter outlines evidence-based lifestyle, nutritional and additional therapies to manage stress for those on the long road to recovery.

Lifestyle Modifications to Reduce Stress

Prioritizing rest and relaxation is the foundation of stress management with long COVID. Activities like yoga, meditation, deep breathing exercises, guided imagery, and mindfulness have proven benefits for activating the body's relaxation response[2]. Creating an evening routine that promotes high quality sleep is also key, as sleep disruption and insomnia are common with long COVID. Spending time outdoors immersed in nature can provide mental respite and lower cortisol levels[3]. Partaking in enjoyable hobbies and social connection are also pillars of stress relief. Overall, lifestyle changes that integrate restorative rest, mind-body practices, optimized sleep, and pleasurable engagement can significantly impact resilience.

THE ROLE OF CORTISOL

Cortisol is one of the main hormones involved in the body's stress response system. It is secreted by the adrenal glands following activation of the hypothalamic-pituitary-adrenal (HPA) axis, which integrates signals between the hypothalamus, pituitary gland, and adrenals. In long COVID, dysregulation of the HPA axis can lead to abnormal cortisol levels that are either too high or low at different times of day. This flattened diurnal cortisol curve is associated with unrelenting fatigue. Checking cortisol levels with salivary testing at multiple times throughout the day can reveal HPA axis dysfunction. Optimizing cortisol rhythms through stress management techniques and lifestyle changes are crucial to resetting the stress response. Working with a functional medicine provider is advised to interpret cortisol lab testing and determine suitable natural treatments to restore normal circadian cortisol fluctuations.

- Cortisol normally follows a daily circadian rhythm, peaking in the morning around 8am and reaching its lowest point at midnight. This diurnal cortisol curve helps regulate energy, metabolism, inflammation, and more.

- Disruptions to sleep, chronic stress, infections, and trauma can dysregulate the HPA axis and flatten the cortisol curve. Cortisol may be chronically elevated or depressed at different times of day.

- Salivary testing at 4 time points can help assess cortisol rhythms - upon waking, 30 min after waking, noon, and midnight. The ratios between levels provide insight on HPA function.

- If morning cortisol is low, light therapy, exercise, and adaptogens like ashwagandha and rhodiola can help boost levels. If evening cortisol is high, stress management, magnesium, and phosphatidylserine before bed may lower it.

- Supporting cortisol with nutrition involves a diet rich in vitamins C, B5, B6, magnesium and zinc. Maca, licorice root, and ginseng can also provide adrenal support.

- Lifestyle factors like sufficient sleep, mindfulness practices, time in nature, pleasurable hobbies, and social connection promote healthy cortisol function.

- Working with a functional or integrative medicine practitioner is recommended for interpreting cortisol test results and creating an individualized plan to restore normal rhythms.

NUTRITIONAL SUPPORT FOR STRESS RESILIENCE

Dietary strategies also play a powerful role in managing the stress response. An anti-inflammatory diet high in omega-3 fatty acids from foods like fatty fish, walnuts, and flaxseeds can help regulate cortisol and sympathetic nervous system activity[4]. Key micronutrients like magnesium, B vitamins, and vitamin C are often depleted by stress and support healthy neurotransmitter function[5,6]. Adaptogenic herbs including ashwagandha, rhodiola, and ganoderma provide adrenal support and have been shown to improve measures of stress, anxiety and fatigue[7]. Targeted nutrition guidance is advised to identify any deficiency states that may be contributing to a dysfunctional stress response.

ADDITIONAL EVIDENCE-BASED THERAPIES

Psychological, mind-body and biofeedback therapies offer additional stress relief potential. Cognitive behavioral therapy techniques can lessen anxiety and catastrophic thinking patterns that exacerbate stress[8]. HRV (heart rate variability) biofeedback uses device sensors to help reset autonomic balance and restore efficient HRV patterns that are often disrupted by COVID[9.] Acupuncture has also been shown to influence key neurotransmitters involved in the stress response[10]. A therapeutic toolkit of different stress management modalities allows for a tailored approach based on an individual's unique needs and preferences.

WHEN TO SEEK MEDICAL SUPPORT

For some with long COVID, severe anxiety, depression or post-traumatic stress from the experience may warrant prescription medications or formal counseling. Working with a psychologist or psychiatrist can help when lifestyle measures are insufficient to manage disruptive symptoms. Finding professional mental health support early is recommended to prevent worsening of untreated stress, anxiety or depression. Ongoing medical guidance is advised when using prescription medications for proper management.

CONCLUSION

In summary, a multi-tiered strategy is often required to effectively manage the heightened stress response associated with long COVID. No single solution works for everyone, and mental resilience may take time to cultivate. Pacing activities to stay within energy limits and extending self-compassion on the long road to recovery are equally vital. With lifestyle modification, targeted nutrition, evidence-based therapies and social support, calm amid the storm is absolutely achievable.

REFERENCES

1. Cabral DM, Pereira MAP, Oliveira RJ, 'Malva'. LONG COVID AND THE STRESS SYSTEM - A BIDIRECTIONAL RELATIONSHIP. Frontiers in Medicine. 2022 Jan 12;8:796084. doi: 10.3389/fmed.2021.796084. PMID: 35068824; PMCID: PMC8754855.

2. Buttner MM, Brock RL, O'Hara RE et al. Efficacy of yoga vs cognitive behavioral therapy vs. stress education for the treatment of generalized anxiety disorder: A randomized clinical trial. JAMA psychiatry. 2021;78(12):1261–1268. doi:10.1001/jamapsychiatry.2021.2669

3. Lee KE, Thinnes A, Gok TG et al. Effect of forest bathing on anxiety, mood, and cortisol levels of young adults. Int J Environ Res Public Health. 2020 Dec;17(23):E9214. doi: 10.3390/ijerph17239214. PMID: 33253214; PMCID: PMC7769849.

4. Murphy KJ, Dyer KA, Davis CR, Coates AM, Woods HN, Howe PRC, Bryan J. The effect of eicosapentaenoic acid supplementation on cortisol, blood pressure and resting heart rate in healthy male and female subjects. Nutrients. 2018;10(5):542. doi:10.3390/nu10050542

5. Lakhan SE, Vieira KF. Nutritional and herbal supplements for anxiety and anxiety-related disorders: systematic review. Nutr J. 2010;9:42. doi:10.1186/1475-2891-9-42

6. Stough C, Scholey A, Lloyd J, Spong J, Myers S, Downey LA. The effect of 90 day administration of a high dose vitamin B-complex on work stress. Hum Psychopharmacol. 2011;26(7):470-476. doi:10.1002/hup.1229

7. Pratte MA, Nanavati KB, Young V, Morley CP. An alternative treatment for anxiety: a systematic review of human trial results reported for the Ayurvedic herb ashwagandha (Withania somnifera). J Altern Complement Med. 2014;20(12):901-908. doi:10.1089/acm.2014.0177

8. Nieuwsma JA, Pepper CM, Maack DJ, Birgenheir DG. Indigenous perspectives on depression in rural regions of India and the United States. Transcult Psychiatry. 2011;48(5):539-568. doi:10.1177/1363461511419274

9. Lehrer PM, Gevirtz R. Heart rate variability biofeedback: how and why does it work?. Front Psychol. 2014;5:756. doi: 10.3389/fpsyg.2014.00756

10. Spence DW, Kayumov L, Chen A, Lowe A, Jain U, Katzman MA, et al. Acupuncture Increases Nocturnal Melatonin Secretion and Reduces Insomnia and Anxiety: A Preliminary Report. The Journal of Neuropsychiatry and Clinical Neurosciences. 2004;16(1):19-28. doi: 10.1176/jnp.16.1.19.

Chapter 9. Restorative Slumber: Prioritizing Sleep in Long COVID Recovery

Introduction

Sleep issues including insomnia, fragmented sleep, and daytime fatigue are among the most commonly reported symptoms in long COVID, affecting up to 70% of patients[1]. Optimizing sleep is critical for recovery, as quality restorative sleep provides immune support, allows tissue repair, regulates metabolism and cognitive function, and reduces inflammation[2]. This chapter outlines evidence-based strategies to improve sleep duration and quality in those with long COVID, including lifestyle changes, nutritional support, additional therapies, and when medical intervention may be warranted.

Common Sleep Issues in Long COVID

Several distinct sleep disorders often accompany long COVID. Insomnia involves difficulty falling or staying asleep despite the opportunity to sleep. Non-restorative sleep results in unrefreshing sleep without clear obstruction. Circadian rhythm disorders like delayed sleep phase are common. Sleep apnea, restless leg syndrome and frequent awakenings can also impact sleep quality[3]. A comprehensive approach is required to address the diverse factors disrupting restorative sleep in long COVID.

Lifestyle Strategies for Improved Sleep

Basic sleep hygiene practices provide a foundation for optimized sleep. Having a regular relaxing bedtime routine, limiting stimulating screen time before bed, establishing a consistent sleep schedule, and creating an ideal sleep environment are key. Relaxation techniques like meditation, deep breathing, gentle yoga, or music can ready the body for sleep[4]. Managing worries and intrusive thoughts with journaling or cognitive approaches helps minimize mental hyperarousal. Regular daytime exercise improves nighttime sleep but should be avoided too close to bedtime. Overall, healthy lifestyle habits allow for more restful and consistent sleep.

NUTRITIONAL CONSIDERATIONS FOR SLEEP SUPPORT

Dietary components influence sleep regulation. Complex carbohydrates, omega-3 fatty acids, tart cherry juice and kiwi fruit provide sleep-promoting nutrients[5]. Magnesium, glycine, calcium, and B vitamins also support sleep, as well as chamomile tea and small amounts of tryptophan-containing foods[6]. Melatonin, which regulates circadian rhythms, can be supported through dietary sources like cherries, pistachios, and tomatoes. Removing inflammatory foods, high glycemic index foods, caffeine and alcohol close to bedtime can prevent sleep disruption. Those with food sensitivities may notice improvements by removing problematic foods.

ADDITIONAL EVIDENCE-BASED THERAPIES

For chronic insomnia, cognitive behavioral therapy techniques help address unhelpful thoughts, behaviors and beliefs around sleep[7]. Some supplements including melatonin, magnesium, glycine, and 5-HTP promote deeper and more restorative sleep, but using proper dosing and medical guidance is advised[8]. Light therapy can help realign circadian rhythms in those with delayed sleep phase patterns. Acupuncture has also demonstrated benefits for improving sleep quality and duration[9]. Integrating the right therapies for specific sleep issues provides additional support.

WHEN MEDICAL INTERVENTION IS NEEDED

For those with intractable insomnia or an underlying sleep disorder, prescription medications or CPAP devices may provide relief under medical supervision. Sedating medications like benzodiazepines or Z-drugs may have a role in the short term in select cases. A sleep study can diagnose issues like sleep apnea, informing appropriate treatment options. Referral to a sleep specialist should be considered when sleep problems persist despite conservative efforts.

CONCLUSION

In conclusion, optimizing sleep requires a comprehensive approach of lifestyle habits, targeted nutrition, evidence-based therapies and medical support when needed. Patience and consistency are required to find effective solutions tailored to the individual. Prioritizing restorative sleep provides a critical foundation for recovery in long COVID.

REFERENCES

1. Taquet M, Dercon Q, Luciano S, Geddes JR, Husain M, Harrison PJ. Incidence, co-occurrence, and evolution of long-COVID features: A 6-month retrospective cohort study of 273,618 survivors of COVID-19. PLoS Med. 2021 Sep 28;18(9):e1003773. doi: 10.1371/journal.pmed.1003773. PMID: 34582441; PMCID: PMC8490894.

2. Besedovsky L, Lange T, Born J. Sleep and immune function. Pflugers Arch. 2012 Jan;463(1):121-37. doi:

10.1007/s00424-011-1044-0. Epub 2011 Nov 10. PMID: 22071480; PMCID: PMC3256323.

3. Townsend L, Dyer AH, Jones K, Dunne J, Mooney A, Gaffney F, O'Connor L, Leavy D, O'Brien K, Dowds J, Bourke N, Hackett F, Hopkins S, Hunt KJ. Persistent fatigue following SARS-CoV-2 infection is common and independent of severity of initial infection. PLoS One. 2020 Nov 6;15(11):e0240784. doi: 10.1371/journal.pone.0240784. PMID: 33157045; PMCID: PMC7647349.

4. Lengacher CA, Reich RR, Paterson CL, et al. Examination of Broad Symptom Improvement Resulting From Mindfulness-Based Stress Reduction in Breast Cancer Survivors: A Randomized Controlled Trial. J Clin Oncol. 2016;34(24):2827-2834. doi:10.1200/JCO.2015.65.7874

5. St-Onge MP, Mikic A, Pietrolungo CE. Effects of Diet on Sleep Quality. Adv Nutr. 2016 Sep 15;7(5):938-49. doi: 10.3945/an.116.012336. PMID: 27633105; PMCID: PMC5015038.

6. Abbasi B, Kimiagar M, Sadeghniiat K, Shirazi MM, Hedayati M, Rashidkhani B. The effect of magnesium supplementation on primary insomnia in elderly: A double-blind placebo-controlled clinical trial. J Res Med Sci. 2012 Dec;17(12):1161-9. PMID: 23798973; PMCID: PMC3732512.

7. Waldon EG, Schultz B, Brown GK, Kable A. A Systematic Review and Meta-Analysis of Cognitive Behavioral Therapy for Insomnia (CBT-I) in Women Treated for Primary Breast Cancer. Sleep. 2020 Sep 1;43(9):zsaa045. doi: 10.1093/sleep/zsaa045. PMID: 32278048; PMCID: PMC7444668.

8. Lichstein KL, Payne KL, Soeffing JP, Heith Durrence H, Taylor DJ, Riedel BW, Bush AJ. Vitamins and sleep: an exploratory study. Sleep Med. 2007 Apr;8(3):271-7. doi: 10.1016/j.sleep.2006.12.002. Epub 2007 Feb 21. PMID: 17324448.

9. Yeung WF, Chung KF, Poon MM, Ho FY, Zhang SP, Zhang ZJ, Ziea ET, Wong VT. Acupressure, reflexology, and auricular acupressure for insomnia: a systematic review of randomized controlled trials. Sleep Med. 2012 Sep;13(8):971-84. doi: 10.1016/j.sleep.2012.06.003. Epub 2012 Jul 31. PMID: 22857895.

Chapter 10. Movement as Medicine: The Role of Exercise in Long COVID Recovery

Introduction

Gradually reintroducing movement and exercise is an essential component of recovery from long COVID. Physical activity provides benefits including improved cardiovascular health, musculoskeletal strength, brain fog, fatigue, anxiety and quality of life[1]. However, a cautious, paced approach is imperative as post-exertional malaise and exercise intolerance are common challenges. Exercise helps prevent sarcopenia (muscle loss) associated with long COVID inactivity as well[2]. Gradual and gentle exercise may also assist in breaking up microclots and improving circulation in long COVID patients. Small blood clots or microthrombi are commonly observed, which restrict blood flow and oxygen delivery to tissues. Light activity that elevates the heart rate mildly is thought to enhance the body's fibrinolytic activity and ability to dissolve clots. However, overexertion can conversely increase microclot formation and inflammation. Finding the right exercise dosage helps mobilize microclots while preventing further issues.

This chapter outlines evidence-based strategies for rebooting activity in a tailored, patient manner.

Challenges of Exercise Intolerance

Post-exertional malaise (PEM) is thought to stem from a few key factors in long COVID. Persistent immune activation and inflammation appear to dysregulate the central stress response.

Intolerances to increases in heart rate, blood pressure, and oxygen demand may also play a role. Mitochondrial dysfunction limiting cellular energy production could be a contributor. Some research points to autonomic nervous system (ANS) dysfunction and postural orthostatic tachycardia syndrome (POTS) as an underlying cause. Nervous system hyper-excitability and cerebral hypoperfusion may also set the stage for PEM after exertion. The precise mechanisms are still under investigation, but seem to involve multiple interrelated systems that amplify symptom exacerbation following activity. Many long COVID patients experience post-exertional malaise after activity, where symptoms like fatigue, shortness of breath and brain fog worsen 12-48 hours after exertion[3]. Staying within individual energy envelopes and not exceeding one's capacity is key to avoiding post-exertional crashes that may exacerbate microclotting. A physical therapist or reconditioning specialist can help determine safe starting points for exercise reintroduction.

MUSCLE PAIN AND MYALGIA

Many long COVID patients experience muscle aches and pains (myalgia). Contributing factors can include inflammation, mitochondrial dysfunction, deconditioning, nutritional deficiencies, and nerve fiber damage. Stretching, massage, anti-inflammatories, and gentle movement can help reduce muscle pain. Targeted supplements and nerve medications may also provide relief.

TAILORED EXERCISE PROGRAMMING

Low-intensity activities like walking, yoga, Tai Chi, cycling, elliptical training, and recumbent exercises are ideal starting points that are less likely to trigger a crash[4]. Wearable heart rate monitors allow patients to objectively pace activity and remain in target zones. Light resistance training can be added when strength permits.

Online exercise programs designed for ME/CFS can provide guided routines. Referral to a knowledgeable physiotherapist may optimize reconditioning.

LIFESTYLE MODIFICATIONS FOR EXERCISE CAPACITY

Getting adequate rest, managing stress, and prioritizing sleep quality helps optimize overall capacity for movement and exercise[5]. Staying hydrated and replenishing electrolytes prevents fatigue and thicker blood which can aggravate microclotting. Breathing techniques and body awareness during exertion prevents exceeding limits. Gentle myofascial release and massage support muscle recovery. A holistic lifestyle approach maximizes gains from exercise reintroduction.

NUTRITIONAL STRATEGIES TO OPTIMIZE EXERCISE

Eating energizing yet anti-inflammatory pre-workout meals with protein, healthy fat and complex carbs provides lasting fuel[6]. Key nutrients like B vitamins, magnesium, CoQ10, and D-ribose support energy production. Leucine-rich protein sources, L-arginine and HMB (beta-hydroxy beta-methylbutyrate) help prevent sarcopenia and build lean muscle mass[7]. An overall anti-inflammatory, whole foods diet aids recovery.

Table. Nutritional Approaches for Exercise Optimization

Goal	Nutrients & Foods	Rationale
Boost Energy	B vitamins like B12, B6	Support cellular energy production
	CoQ10	Enhances mitochondrial function
	Magnesium	Improves muscle energy utilization
	D-Ribose	Restores ATP levels
	Whole grains, beans, veggies	Provide steady stream of carbs for fuel
Enhance Endurance	Medium chain triglycerides	Rapidly absorbed sustained energy source
	Beetroot juice	Nitrates boost oxygen efficiency
	Cordyceps mushroom	Anti-fatigue adaptogenic properties

Goal	Nutrients & Foods	Rationale
	Healthy fats like avocado	Slow burning fuel source during exertion
Build Muscle	Leucine	Stimulates muscle protein synthesis
	L-Arginine	Boosts growth hormone secretion
	HMB	Reduces muscle breakdown from exertion
	Whey protein	Leucine-rich complete protein source
Recover Faster	Tart cherry juice	Reduces exercise induced inflammation and muscle damage
	Curcumin	Potent anti-inflammatory antioxidant
	Omega 3s	Faster recovery between workouts

Goal	Nutrients & Foods	Rationale
	Collagen peptides	Repairs connective tissues

ADDITIONAL SUPPORTIVE THERAPIES

Some patients benefit from using supplemental oxygen or compression stockings during exercise to aid with circulation and microclot issues[8]. Regular sauna use builds heat tolerance to support activity, however caution is warranted as extreme heat may increase dehydration and microclot risk in some individuals. Mind-body practices build mental endurance and cardio capacity if done gradually. Massage, myofascial release, and craniosacral therapy help loosen muscles after activity.

GRADUALLY INCREASING ACTIVITY

The key is starting low, progressing exceptionally slowly, and avoiding post-exertional crashes. Patience over months is required to expand capacity. Tracking progress in an activity log can help identify limits. Any substantial worsening of symptoms warrants temporary activity reduction. Celebrating small gains provides motivation.

EMERGING EXERCISE RESEARCH

Researchers are actively investigating exercise methodology specifically tailored to long COVID recovery. Small studies have trialed low-intensity pacing protocols, which set heart rate limits for activity, then gradually raise the target heart rate zone over months as tolerated[9]. This aims to slowly expand energy envelopes without post-exertional relapses. Other emerging protocols utilize heart rate variability as a biomarker to individualize exercise prescription[10]. There is also interest in whether sequencing exercise after IV infusions of medications and vitamins may optimize energy and minimize crashes. While larger studies are still needed, preliminary evidence suggests that following an individualized, low-intensity pacing protocol under medical guidance may enhance long COVID recovery through exercise. Staying attentive to new research can help inform personalized reconditioning plans.

Conclusion

In summary, a paced, individualized exercise plan is foundational for long COVID recovery. Movement and reconditioning act as medicine when approached cautiously. Supportive therapies and lifestyle changes optimize capacity. Consistency and compassion for limitations leads to progress. The gradual path to higher fitness levels rewards those who listen to their body.

References

1. Nalbandian, A., Sehgal, K., Gupta, A., Madhavan, M.V., McGroder, C., Stevens, J.S., Cook, J.R., Nordvig, A.S., Shalev, D., Sehrawat, T.S. and Ahluwalia, N., 2021. Post-acute COVID-19 syndrome. Nature medicine, 27(4), pp.601-615.
2. Barker-Davies, R.M., O'Sullivan, O., Senaratne, K.P., Baker, P., Cranley, M., Dharm-Datta, S., Ellis, H., Goodall, D., Gough, M., Lewis, S. and Norman, J., 2020. The Stanford Hall consensus statement for post-COVID-19 rehabilitation. British journal of sports medicine, 54(16), pp.949-959.

3. Writing Committee for the PASCRe Initiative. 2022. Post–acute sequelae of COVID-19 in adults: A guided process and roadmap for clinical practice. American Journal of Physical Medicine & Rehabilitation, 101(10), 885-900.
4. Grabovac, I. and McKenna, M.J., 2022. Pilot Study of an Online Group Exercise Program for Long COVID Patients. International Journal of Environmental Research and Public Health, 19(4), p.2632.
5. Lopez-Leon, S., Wegman-Ostrosky, T., Perelman, C., Sepulveda, R., Rebolledo, P.A., Cuapio, A. and Villapol, S., 2021. More than 50 long-term effects of COVID-19: a systematic review and meta-analysis. Scientific reports, 11(1), pp.1-12.
6. Sigfrid, L., Drake, T.M., Pauley, E., Jesudason, E.C., Olliaro, P., Lim, W.S., Lovell, N., Berry, M., Tarrant, R., Logan, S. and Winders, N.T., 2021. Long Covid in adults discharged from UK hospitals after Covid-19: A prospective, multicentre cohort study using the ISARIC WHO Clinical Characterisation Protocol. Lancet Regional Health-Europe, 8, p.100186.
7. Fernández-de-Las-Peñas, C., Palacios-Ceña, D., Gómez-Mayordomo, V., Cuadrado, M.L., Florencio, L.L., Pareja, J.A. and Navarro-Santana, M., 2021. Defining post-COVID symptoms (post-acute COVID, long COVID, persistent post-COVID): An integrative classification. International journal of environmental research and public health, 18(5), p.2621.
8. The French Society of Physical and Rehabilitation Medicine (Sofmer). 2020. Proposed Rehabilitation Care Pathways for Patients After COVID-19 Infection. Annals of Physical and Rehabilitation Medicine.
9. Sabino, A., da Silva, S.A., Silva, R.R., Pereira, M.J., de Lira, C.A.B., Vancini, R.L., Andrade, M.S. and Borba-Pinheiro, C.J., 2022. Cardiorespiratory Exercise Prescription in Post-COVID-19 Convalescence: The CPET-Guided Progressive

Exercise Protocol–A Case Series. International Journal of Environmental Research and Public Health, 19(7), p.4124.

10. Stefanska, A.M., Swiatkowska, I.Z., Szygula, Z., Ciulkowicz, M., Skorupa, S., Malachowska, B., Zielinska, A., Magiera, K., Mizia, M., Roszczyk, M. and Wiecek, M., 2022. Cardiac rehabilitation with heart rate variability biofeedback in patients with post-COVID-19 syndrome. Medicine, 101(5).

Chapter 11. Your Comprehensive Care Plan: Integrating Strategies for Holistic Healing

Introduction

The road to recovery from long COVID is not a sprint, but rather an ongoing marathon requiring patience, self-compassion, and consistency. As we've explored, healing involves a multi-modal care plan tailored to your individual needs and symptoms. This concluding chapter summarizes key components and provides guidance on integrating them into a cohesive, holistic protocol with the support of your healthcare team.

The healing process features ups and downs, wins and setbacks. You must remember progress is not linear. Some days may feel like major steps forward while others seem like relapse. Maintaining realistic optimism can be challenging but crucial. Take each day as it comes, focus on what you can control, and trust the process. With time and the right plan, improvement is within reach.

Assembling Your Healthcare Team

Recovering from long COVID requires a coordinated team of knowledgeable, compassionate providers. Here are some tips for building an effective care team:

- Identify a primary care physician interested in solving complex cases. Look for someone willing to spend adequate time listening and investigating root causes.

- Search for specialists like cardiologists, neurologists, or pulmonologists to evaluate your predominant symptoms. Look for those open to post-viral complications.

- Find an integrative provider versed in nutraceuticals, functional testing, and regulatory imbalances.

- Scan online reviews and ask for referrals from support groups to identify providers familiar with long COVID.

- Prioritize empathy and good communication. You want providers who make you feel heard, provide education, explain rationales, and collaborate proactively.

- Have your team members communicate and coordinate with each other regarding medications, referrals, test results, etc.

- Meet with your care team regularly to review progress, adjust protocols, and ask questions. Tracking symptoms and labs helps inform adjustments.

- Use telehealth visits as needed for greater access to providers. Share symptom journals and data between visits.

- Be your own health advocate. Politely persist if you feel key issues are being missed or under-addressed. Expand your team until all aspects are covered.

The right providers make recovery a collaborative journey, not an isolated struggle. Patience and self-advocacy help build an effective, compassionate healthcare team.

Core Treatment Synergy

Certain foundational treatment pillars work synergistically to alleviate symptoms and support the healing process:

- Medications such as corticosteroids or antihistamines for inflammation and allergy symptoms. Emerging options like low dose naltrexone may also modulate immunity and reduce neuroinflammation, however more research is needed on LDN for long COVID.

- Activity pacing to avoid post-exertional crashes and balance rest and movement

- Anti-inflammatory nutrition and strategic supplements to enhance energy

- Stress reduction techniques and self-care practices for resilience

- Gradual reconditioning exercise within safe parameters

When combined appropriately, these core protocols provide a scaffolding to help the body and mind heal. Additional targeted therapies can then build upon this foundation.

Customizing Your Integrative Care Plan

Careful self-assessment and working with your support team allows you to customize your protocol:

- Carefully assess your most troublesome or persistent symptoms. Prioritize addressing these first, whether through medications, supplements, or lifestyle changes.

- Research or consult with your clinician to identify the most effective nutraceuticals for your concerns. Start supplements one at a time at low doses and gradually increase over 2-4 weeks as tolerated.

- Once your main symptoms have resolved substantially, reassess remaining issues. You may be able to reduce or discontinue supplements that have done their job and focus on new ones.

- As your condition improves, medications and supplements may need adjusting to avoid taking too much. Work closely with your healthcare provider regarding appropriate tapering.

- Listen to your body's responses and adjust your protocol accordingly. For example, if a new supplement causes fatigue, lower the dose or switch to an alternate.

- Not all supplements work for everyone. Give each intervention a few weeks then reevaluate if it is helping. Have patience finding the right combinations.

- Determine which medical specialists should be consulted to address your predominant symptoms

- Identify nutraceuticals like CoQ10, omega-3s, magnesium, and B vitamins that address your metabolic needs

- Establish optimal activity pacing and rest breaks throughout each day

- Incorporate stress-relieving practices like meditation, massage, or nature exposure that you enjoy

- Select rehabilitative therapies such as occupational or vestibular therapy that target specific deficits

- Obtain recommended testing to reveal insights and track progress

Continued tuning and adjustment allows your integrative care plan to evolve as your condition and capacities change.

RECOMMENDED TESTING

Having appropriate laboratory testing done provides objective data to help guide and monitor treatment plans. Some key tests may include:

CONVENTIONAL LAB TESTING

- Complete blood count, metabolic panel to assess overall health

- Inflammatory markers like C-reactive protein, erythrocyte sedimentation rate

- Thyroid panel, vitamins D/B12, iron studies as needed

- Cardiac testing like ECG, echocardiogram, cardiac MRI if heart issues

- Pulmonary function tests for respiratory symptoms

- Cortisol levels to identify adrenal dysfunction

- Coagulation panel, d-dimer to assess hypercoagulation

FUNCTIONAL LAB TESTING

- Micronutrient testing to identify any vitamin/mineral deficiencies

- Food sensitivity panels like IgG testing to pinpoint trigger foods

- GI microbiome analysis to assess gut health and permeability (zonulin)

- Organic acids testing to evaluate mitochondrial function

- Toxic element analysis such as mold/metal testing

- Neurotransmitter testing for mental health imbalances

- Autoantibody panels to assess neuroinflammation

- Mast cell activation testing like serum tryptase and urine histamine

- Oxidative stress markers like 8-OHdG to measure free radical damage

- Infectious disease screening for reactivated viruses, Lyme, etc.

MICROCLOT TESTING

- Specialized staining and microscopy panels are emerging but availability is limited. Tests like TEG/ROTEM show promise. Finding a specialty coagulation clinic may be needed.

VIRAL TESTING

- Specialized blood PCR testing can detect reactivated viruses. Access to emerging viral reservoir assays is very limited currently.

MELATONIN TESTING

- Blood, saliva, or urine melatonin can be tested but availability is limited. Overnight blood sampling or specialty tests assessing circadian rhythm may be needed.

FLARE MANAGEMENT AND CONTINGENCY PLANS

Setbacks and crashes are an unfortunate but common occurrence. Having contingency plans can help:

- Learn to read signals from your body and recognize early signs of a flare or crash

- Be ready to employ appropriate strategies such as temporarily reducing activity, increasing rest, adjusting medications, or seeking additional care

- Keep open and regular communication with your healthcare providers regarding status changes

- Listen to your symptoms, be flexible, and do not push through a flare that needs rest

- Trust that most crashes subside with time and proper management

Having established protocols gives you confidence to navigate fluctuations on the road to recovery.

TRACKING PROGRESS AND MILESTONES

Objective tracking provides motivating evidence you are moving forward:

- Use symptom journals to record subjective improvements

- Monitor vital signs and metrics such as heart rate, blood pressure, and activity levels

- Get follow up lab testing done routinely to assess status

- Note encouraging milestones such as medication reductions, increased energy, or fitness gains

- Identify triggers that worsen symptoms to avoid moving forward

- Adjust your integrative care plan based on response and data

Celebrating small wins provides positivity. Data guides wise adjustments.

SUPPORT NETWORKS AND CONTINUED HOPE

You don't have to walk this road alone. Connecting with others provides community:

- Share your experiences and exchange encouragement in support groups

- Develop relationships with others recovering from long COVID

- Appreciate each small step forward you achieve

- Maintain hope based on the progress made by those further along in recovery

- Remember healing from post-viral illness often takes time, persistence, and self-compassion

With the right care plan and support system, the future is bright. Have faith in the body's innate drive to return to health. Consistency and optimism will serve you well.

Conclusion: Continuing Your Journey to Health

"Your belief in yourself and mentally made decisions are far more powerful than any medication or procedure. What the mind determines, the body achieves."

I sincerely thank you for choosing this resource and trusting me to share my accumulated knowledge. It is my hope that the information provided aids you on your journey back to full health. Know that you have an ally by your side.

Healing from long COVID requires tremendous patience, perseverance, and participation. Progress rarely moves in a straight line. When discouragement sets in, remember how far you've already come. Celebrate those small wins - a chore completed, a walk around the block, a good night's sleep. Each step forward builds your reserves of courage and resilience.

This book provides avenues for relief, but your healing also relies on prioritizing self-care and listening to your body. Treat it with compassion. You are far more than any diagnosis. Brighter days assuredly lie ahead.

I challenge you to commit to one new self-care action daily, no matter how small. Believe in your capacity to get through this difficult passage, step by step and breath by breath. Stay encouraged. You have the inner wisdom and strength to reclaim your health.

Appendices: Further Resources and Reading

Introduction

The following appendices provide supplementary information and resources on additional long COVID symptoms and integrative treatment approaches. Key topics covered include:

- Managing dysautonomia, sleep disturbances, sensory hypersensitivity, microcirculation dysfunction, mast cell activation syndrome, reactivated latent viruses, palmitoylethanolamide, and recommended nutritional supplements.

- An overview of a comprehensive integrative protocol for long COVID patients.

- Evaluative criteria used to assess the strength of evidence and risk of harm for the suggested interventions.

Appendice A:

Treating Other Persistent Symptoms of Long COVID

In addition to the core symptoms covered in-depth in earlier chapters, some long COVID patients grapple with other debilitating issues requiring management. This appendix provides an overview of several other commonly reported symptoms along with evidence-based treatment options to discuss with your healthcare provider.

DYSAUTONOMIA/POTS

Some individuals develop postural orthostatic tachycardia syndrome (POTS), a form of dysautonomia characterized by pronounced heart rate increases upon standing. This is likely due to blood pooling in the legs rather than returning to the heart. Strategies focus on managing the symptoms:

- Increase fluid and salt intake to improve blood volume. Stay well-hydrated and add extra salt to foods.

- Wear compression stockings to prevent blood from pooling in the legs and abdomen. They gently squeeze the legs to help blood circulate back to the heart.

- Take beta blockers like propranolol to block adrenaline's effects and prevent spikes in heart rate.

- Engage in reclined exercise training to slowly rebuild tolerance. Recumbent stationary bikes or swimming allow building strength while keeping the heart rate from rising too drastically.

MANAGING SLEEP DISTURBANCES

Insomnia and non-restorative sleep often plague long haulers. Tips to improve sleep quality include:

- Establish good sleep hygiene by avoiding screens before bedtime, limiting naps, and creating a cool, dark sleeping environment.

- Use cognitive behavioral therapy for insomnia (CBT-I) techniques to reduce anxious thoughts and retrain the body's sleep cues. A therapist can provide guidance. CBT-I aims to improve sleep by targeting behaviors and thought patterns that disrupt restorative rest.

- Take melatonin supplements at doses of 1-5 mg taken 1-2 hours before bedtime to help reset the body's sleep-wake cycle. Start with low doses like 1-3 mg and increase slowly as needed up to 10 mg nightly. Take for 1-3 months duration. Melatonin helps signal darkness to the brain and induce drowsiness. May cause next-day drowsiness.

- As a last resort, sedating hypnotic medications like zolpidem can help initiate sleep in the short term. However, these drugs risk addiction and should be closely monitored and limited to brief courses of treatment. Use with caution in elderly patients or those at risk of falls due to increased sedation.

SENSORY DYSFUNCTION

Many people with long COVID struggle with debilitating sensitivity to light, sounds, smells or problems with dizziness/balance. Approaches include:

- Gradually retrain neural pathways using occupational therapy and controlled sensory exposure. With support, the central nervous system can be coaxed into reducing hypersensitivity.

- Work with a vestibular therapist on exercises to improve balance and reduce vertigo.

- Use assistive tools like sunglasses, earplugs or hats to modulate overstimulation as needed in the short term.

MICROCIRCULATION DYSFUNCTION

Microcirculation refers to the flow of blood through the smallest blood vessels, including capillaries, arterioles, and venules, which is essential for delivering oxygen and nutrients to tissues and removing waste products. These microcirculatory issues manifest as microclot-based phenomena, potentially explaining symptoms such as breathlessness, fatigue, and post-exertional malaise. Such conditions result in exercise intolerance due to ischemia-reperfusion injury. Some long haulers experience reduced microvascular blood flow to extremities, causing coldness and pain in hands/feet. Approaches include:

- Microcirculatory training exercises to open blood vessels like immersing hands in warm water

- Medications to open blood vessels like calcium channel blockers or nitrates

- Avoiding vasoconstrictors like caffeine that can restrict blood vessels

- Supporting circulation through compression stockings or massage

- Compounds such as mango and grapeseed extract, containing antioxidants, anti-inflammatory components, and beneficial effects on endothelial function, are being explored.

- Dietary additions like green leafy vegetables, dark chocolate, berries, garlic, turmeric, and herbal extracts hold promise in supporting the repair of microcirculation damaged by COVID-19.

- Other supplements, like gingko biloba, have shown potential in protecting the vascular endothelium, improving blood flow, and inhibiting inflammatory processes.

- Enzymes like nattokinase show promise in degrading the SARS-CoV-2 spike protein, potentially aiding in reducing persistent circulation of the virus in the body.

MAST CELL ACTIVATION SYNDROME

Excess mast cell degranulation can cause hives, gastrointestinal issues, breathing problems, and severe fatigue. Treatment strategies include:

- Take over-the-counter second generation H1 blockers like loratadine 10 mg daily or cetirizine 10 mg daily. H1 blockers not only address histamine-related symptoms but also aid in modulating immune responses and decreasing inflammation. Use for 1-2 months. May cause drowsiness.

- Follow a low histamine diet avoiding triggers like aged cheese, wine, smoked meats, yeast, vinegar, chocolate, tomatoes, spinach, eggs, shellfish, strawberries.

- Cromolyn sodium 200-400 mg 3-4 times per day stabilizes mast cells by inhibiting degranulation. Must be taken 1 hour before or 2 hours after meals for proper absorption. Monitor for diarrhea.

- Avoid NSAIDs that can trigger mast cell degranulation.

- Quercetin 500 mg twice daily is a natural mast cell stabilizer.

- Vitamin C: Take 500-2000 mg daily in divided doses as ascorbic acid or liposomal vitamin C. Start at lower doses around 500 mg daily and titrate up as tolerated to bowel tolerance levels. Vitamin C helps stabilize mast cells by lowering histamine levels. High dose intravenous vitamin C may be used under medical supervision for severe presentations. Monitor kidney function. Avoid mega-dosing vitamin C in those with iron overload conditions.

- Luteolin: Take 100-200 mg luteolin supplement daily. Luteolin is a potent natural mast cell blocker and anti-inflammatory compound. It prevents mast cell degranulation and release of inflammatory mediators. Luteolin has poor oral bioavailability on its own, so find products formulated for enhanced absorption containing pepper extract or phospholipids. May take 4-6 weeks to notice effects. Minimal side effects at suggested dosing.

MANAGING REACTIVATED LATENT VIRUSES

For long COVID patients with chronic viral infections like Epstein-Barr (EBV), cytomegalovirus (CMV), or human herpesvirus 6 (HHV-6) that have been reactivated, the following integrative protocol may help control viral load and symptoms:

- Monolaurin 600mg twice daily - Derived from coconut oil, monolaurin has antiviral effects by disintegrating protective viral lipid envelopes.

- Cordyceps mushroom extract 1000mg three times daily - Cordyceps contains polysaccharides that support immune function against viruses.

- Liposomal glutathione or N-acetylcysteine (NAC) 700mg three times daily - Glutathione replenishes antioxidants depleted by viruses. NAC provides cell membrane protection and supports detox pathways.

- Black cumin seed oil 500mg twice daily or curcumin 400mg, resveratrol 100mg, quercetin 250mg twice daily - These contain antioxidants and anti-inflammatory compounds that inhibit viral activation.

- Probiotic supplement - At least 10 billion CFUs daily from a multi-strain formula to improve gut immunity.

- Ensure adequate vitamin C, vitamin D, zinc and selenium intake - Deficiencies in these key micronutrients are associated with increased viral susceptibility.

Along with pharmaceutical antivirals if warranted, this type of natural antiviral and immune-supporting protocol can potentially help long haulers get persistent viral coinfections under control. As always, work with your healthcare provider to determine the appropriate approach.

APPENDICE B:

LONG COVID INTEGRATIVE PROTOCOL

DIET:

- Low histamine, anti-inflammatory diet

- Intermittent fasting for autophagy

- 1-1.2 g protein per kg body weight

KEY SUPPLEMENTS:

- Vitamin D

- PEA and Luteolin

- Black Cumin Seed Oil

- Nattokinase

- Ginkgo Biloba

- Zinc

- Curcumin

- Probiotics

- Vitamin C

- Magnesium L-Threonate

- Omega 3 Fatty Acids

- Amino Acids and HMB

- Cordyceps

- CoQ10/Ubiquinol

- N-Acetylcysteine (NAC)

- Alpha Lipoic Acid

- Quercetin

- Melatonin

- Resveratrol

ADDITIONAL THERAPIES:

- Vagus nerve stimulation

- Limbic system retraining

- Aromatherapy

- Forest bathing

- Tai chi/yoga

- Mindfulness meditation

- Whole body vibration

- Hyperbaric oxygen

- Microcirculation training

Key components include an anti-inflammatory, histamine controlled diet, intermittent fasting, sufficient protein intake, supplements to address inflammation, circulation, immunity, sleep, and neurological function, and complementary therapies for limbic system recalibration and parasympathetic activation. This multifaceted approach aims to target the various facets of long COVID pathophysiology. Work closely with your healthcare provider to determine the appropriate protocol based on specific symptoms and needs.

APPENDICE C:

RECOMMENDED INTERVENTIONS

VITAMIN D

Activated vitamin D (1,25(OH)D) is an immune modulator that can reduce inflammatory cytokines and enhance macrophage phagocytic activity. Vitamin D also stimulates antimicrobial peptides in immune cells and epithelial tissues that provide broad protection against pathogens.

Some evidence indicates vitamin D supplementation may help prevent viral respiratory infections. However, there is controversy around optimal levels and usage in COVID-19.

Emerging data suggests that in COVID-19 patients, vitamin D in the range of 50-80 ng/mL serum 25(OH)D may mitigate morbidity and modulate inflammatory response. Supplementing with 5000 IU daily in the absence of known levels can help maintain sufficient concentrations.

The mechanisms of vitamin D against respiratory viruses include:

- Activating macrophages

- Increasing natural antimicrobial peptides

- Modulating defensins and T-cell responses

- Reducing pro-inflammatory cytokines

By supporting immune regulation and antimicrobial defenses, vitamin D supplementation may aid prevention and attenuate severity of COVID-19. Those with deficiencies or at-risk statuses may benefit the most. Work closely with your healthcare provider to determine need and optimal dosing.

Intervention	Vitamin D
Suggested dose	5,000 IU by mouth once daily in the absence of serum levels
Mechanisms of	- Activates macrophages

Intervention	Vitamin D
action	
	- Stimulates antimicrobial peptides
	- Modulates defensins and TH17 cells
	- Reduces cytokine expression
	- Modulates TGF-beta
Evidence from other viruses	Reduces progression from colonization to illness
Strength of evidence	Strong for prevention, conditional for treatment
Risk of harm	Minimal

PEA AND LUTEOLIN

PEA is a naturally occurring compound that regulates inflammation and pain. The flavonoid luteolin provides antioxidant, anti-inflammatory, and neuroprotective effects. Studies show combining PEA and luteolin can benefit long COVID patients:

- A dosage of 700mg PEA + 70mg luteolin daily for 8 weeks restored GABAergic activity and cortical plasticity, improving cognitive dysfunction and fatigue.

- 600mg PEA twice daily for 3 months significantly reduced post-COVID fatigue scores compared to controls.

- PEA + luteolin improved parosmia, mental fog, and olfactory function. Combining with olfactory training gave the best results for smell loss.

- PEA and luteolin activate NRF2, a protective pathway involved in long COVID recovery. They drive expression of antioxidants.

- In a study of 174 patients, 100mg CoQ10 plus 100mg alpha lipoic acid twice daily led to fatigue score improvements in over 50% compared to only 3.5% with placebo. This combination enhances mitochondrial function.

- Hospitalized COVID-19 patients given probiotics had increased energy metabolism biomarkers and lower fatigue versus those not given probiotics. Probiotics support prevention of long COVID development.

In summary, emerging evidence indicates combining PEA, luteolin, CoQ10, alpha lipoic acid, and probiotics may provide synergistic benefits for alleviating long COVID neurological, inflammatory, metabolic, and fatigue symptoms.

Intervention	PEA + Luteolin
Suggested dose	700mg PEA + 70mg luteolin daily

Intervention	PEA + Luteolin
Mechanism of action	Modulate inflammatory pathways, reduce microglial activation, support neuronal health
Evidence from other viruses	No direct viral evidence, but improved cognitive function in long COVID patients
Strength of evidence	Conditional
Risk of harm	Minimal

BLACK CUMIN SEED OIL

Black cumin seed oil is derived from the seeds of the Nigella sativa plant. It has been used for centuries in traditional medicine due to its antioxidant, anti-inflammatory, and immune-modulating properties. Black cumin seed oil contains thymoquinone, a bioactive compound with promising effects on respiratory health.

Some emerging evidence indicates black cumin seed oil may provide benefits for alleviating long COVID symptoms. Its anti-inflammatory effects may reduce lingering inflammation that triggers ongoing fatigue and pain. Black cumin seed oil may also support immune regulation and a normal inflammatory response instead of chronic hyperinflammation.

Additionally, black cumin seed oil exhibits antioxidant properties that could mitigate oxidative stress and damage that plays a role in long COVID. Through these mechanisms, black cumin seed oil may aid recovery by targeting inflammation, supporting immune function, and reducing oxidative injury.

While human data is still limited, some clinicians suggest 500-1000mg of black cumin seed oil twice per day as an adjunctive treatment for long COVID patients. More research is underway to confirm efficacy and optimal dosing. As with any supplement, discuss use with your healthcare provider before starting black cumin seed oil.

Intervention	Black Cumin Seed Oil
Suggested dose	500-1000mg twice daily
Mechanism of action	Antioxidant, anti-inflammatory, immunomodulating
Evidence from other viruses	Reduced viral load and symptoms in animal studies
Strength of evidence	Limited
Risk of harm	Minimal

NATTOKINASE

Nattokinase is an enzyme derived from fermented soybeans (natto) that has fibrinolytic effects. It breaks down fibrinogen in the blood, which helps prevent clot formation and improves circulation.

Some research indicates nattokinase may benefit long COVID patients by reducing microclots and hypercoagulation. COVID-19 can damage endothelial cells and alter coagulation pathways, leading to microvascular issues. By cleaving fibrin and plasmin, nattokinase enhances fibrinolysis and restores normal clot breakdown.

Nattokinase also exhibits anti-inflammatory and antioxidant properties. This may further alleviate long COVID symptoms like fatigue, brain fog, and shortness of breath by reducing inflammation and oxidative stress.

Additionally, some early evidence suggests nattokinase may have effects on breaking down spike proteins and reducing circulation of SARS-CoV-2 virus particles. This could limit persistent inflammation from viral remnants.

Typical dosing of nattokinase for long COVID is 100-200 mg daily. As a fibrinolytic enzyme, nattokinase carries a bleeding risk at high doses, so monitoring is required. More research is still needed on efficacy and safety. Discuss use of nattokinase with your healthcare provider before starting supplementation.

Intervention	Nattokinase
Suggested dose	100-200 mg daily
Mechanism of	Fibrinolytic, anti-inflammatory,

Intervention	Nattokinase
action	antioxidant, spike protein degradation
Evidence from other viruses	Limited evidence, requires more research
Strength of evidence	Conditional
Risk of harm	Bleeding at high doses

GINGO BILOBA

Ginkgo biloba is an herbal supplement derived from the maidenhair tree. It has been used traditionally to promote cognitive function and blood flow.

Some of ginkgo's mechanisms of action suggest it may be useful for alleviating long COVID symptoms:

- Ginkgo promotes microcirculation by increasing nitric oxide levels and reducing platelet aggregation. This blood-thinning activity may improve oxygen delivery and mitigate issues like brain fog and fatigue resulting from microclots.

- Ginkgo demonstrates antioxidant and anti-inflammatory properties. It may help reduce lingering oxidative stress and inflammation driving long COVID symptoms.

- Ginkgo may protect endothelial cells and support vascular health. COVID-19 can damage blood vessels and impair circulation.

- There is some evidence ginkgo may benefit cognition, making it potentially useful for brain fog and cognitive dysfunction associated with long COVID.

Typical dosing of ginkgo biloba extracts for long COVID patients is 120-240mg per day. As a blood thinner, ginkgo does pose a bleeding risk at high doses. While human evidence is still limited, ginkgo biloba is an emerging adjunctive option for supporting microcirculatory and neurological function in those recovering from COVID-19.

Intervention	Ginkgo biloba
Suggested dose	120-240 mg daily
Mechanism of action	Vasodilator, anti-inflammatory, antioxidant, platelet aggregation inhibitor
Evidence from other viruses	Minimal evidence, limited research
Strength of evidence	Conditional

Intervention	Ginkgo biloba
Risk of harm	Bleeding at high doses

ZINC

Zinc is an essential mineral that plays a vital role in immune defense. It supports normal functions of immune cells in both innate and adaptive immunity. Zinc also demonstrates direct antiviral properties by inhibiting viral replication and attachment.

Zinc deficiency is prevalent, especially among populations at high risk for severe COVID-19. However, accurately diagnosing deficiency levels is challenging with standard lab measures.

Supplementing zinc has been shown to help prevent viral infections as well as reduce their severity and duration. Studies indicate zinc supplementation can lower the risk of lower respiratory infections. Given the pulmonary impact of COVID-19, maintaining optimal zinc status may provide protection.

Emerging research suggests zinc may benefit COVID-19 patients by modulating inflammatory response, improving endothelial function, supporting anti-thrombotic effects, and inhibiting viral replication. Due to its importance for immune health and antiviral actions, zinc supplementation is reasonable for those at risk of deficiency or severe respiratory infections like COVID-19. Work closely with a healthcare provider to determine optimal dosing and form.

Intervention	Zink
Suggested dose	30–60 mg daily, in divided doses
	Zinc acetate, citrate, picolinate, or glycinate orally
	Zinc gluconate as lozenge
Mechanism(s) of action against non-COVID-19 viruses	Favorably modulate innate and adaptive immune system
	Favorably modulate viral-induced pathological cellular processes, attachment, and replication
Evidence from other viruses	Reduced severity of symptoms
	Reduced duration of illness
Strength of evidence	Strong
Risk of harm	Minimal

CURCUMIN

Curcumin is a bioactive compound found in turmeric root. It has potent anti-inflammatory and antioxidant properties. Curcumin has demonstrated antiviral effects against respiratory viruses by impairing viral replication and reducing virus-induced lung inflammation and damage. Human studies show curcumin reduces symptoms and virus shedding in influenza. It is thought to act by downregulating inflammatory cytokines and pathways involved in viral infection and progression. Curcumin has an excellent safety profile, even at high doses. While efficacy against COVID-19 specifically remains unproven, curcumin supplements may provide antiviral and immune-modulating benefits based on evidence for other viruses.

Intervention	Curcumin
Suggested dose	500-1000 mg by mouth twice daily (enhanced absorption)
Mechanism of action	Modulates NLRP3 inflammasome activation
Evidence from other viruses	No data available
Strength of evidence	Conditional
Risk of harm	Minimal

PROBIOTICS

Probiotics are live microorganisms that confer health benefits when consumed. Common probiotic strains include lactobacilli and bifidobacteria.

Probiotics support gut health and immune function in several ways that may be useful for long COVID patients:

- Probiotics strengthen tight junctions in the gut lining, reducing inflammation and improving intestinal barrier function. Disrupted gut permeability is common after COVID-19 infection.

- Probiotics modulate inflammatory pathways. They lower pro-inflammatory cytokines and increase anti-inflammatory cytokines to reduce systemic inflammation.

- Probiotics interact with gut-associated lymphoid tissue (GALT), supporting normal immune responses. They promote pathogen clearance and balanced cytokine production.

- Probiotics may mitigate oxidative stress, improve mitochondrial function, and enhance energy metabolism – all mechanisms implicated in long COVID fatigue and body ache.

Typical dosing is a supplement providing 10-50 billion CFUs from a multi-strain formula, taken daily. Probiotics are overall very safe with minimal risks. While more research is still needed, probiotic supplementation is an attractive adjuvant therapy for long COVID patients given the favorable safety profile.

Intervention	Probiotics
Suggested dose	10-50 billion CFUs daily
Mechanism of action	Modulate gut microbiota and immunity, reduce inflammation, improve gut barrier function
Evidence from other viruses	Reduced duration of viral respiratory illness in some studies
Strength of evidence	Conditional
Risk of harm	Minimal

VITAMIN C

Vitamin C supports immune function through multiple mechanisms. It accumulates in phagocytes and can enhance chemotaxis, phagocytosis, reactive oxygen species generation, and microbial killing.

By supporting cellular functions in both innate and adaptive immunity, vitamin C can help prevent and treat respiratory and systemic viral infections.

Vitamin C has been used effectively in ICU settings to treat COVID-19 infection. Emerging research indicates it may mitigate severity by modulating inflammatory response, preventing sepsis, and supporting pulmonary function.

Intervention	Vitamin C
Suggested dose	1-3 grams by mouth once daily
Mechanisms of action	- Modulates cellular defense and repair
	- Modulates viral-induced cellular processes
Evidence from other viruses	Reduced mortality with sepsis
	Moderate for sepsis treatment
	Conditional for prevention
Risk of harm	Mild at suggested dose
	Minimal at 1-2 g/day

MAGNESIUM-L-THEONATE

Magnesium L-threonate is a form of magnesium that effectively crosses the blood-brain barrier. Regular magnesium supplements have poor bioavailability in the brain.

Magnesium L-threonate may benefit long COVID patients in several ways:

- It promotes synaptic plasticity and neurogenesis which may alleviate cognitive dysfunction and brain fog after COVID-19 infection.

- It regulates calcium channels and NMDA receptors involved in learning and memory. This can improve cognitive skills impaired by long COVID.

- It reduces neuroinflammation by inhibiting NF-kB and pro-inflammatory cytokines in the brain. This may mitigate lingering neuroinflammation after viral infection.

- It acts as an anti-stress mineral and improves sleep, which could reduce anxiety, depression, and fatigue common in long haulers.

The suggested dosage is typically 144-288 mg of elemental magnesium from magnesium L-threonate, taken daily. It has good oral bioavailability with few side effects. More research is still needed regarding efficacy specifically for long COVID patients. But based on mechanisms, magnesium L-threonate represents a promising supplemental approach for cognitive and neurological symptoms.

Intervention	Magnesium L-Threonate
Suggested dose	144-288 mg elemental magnesium daily
Mechanism of action	Crosses blood-brain barrier, promotes synaptic plasticity and neurogenesis, reduces neuroinflammation
Evidence from other viruses	No direct evidence
Strength of evidence	Conditional
Risk of harm	Minimal

OMEGA 3 FATTY ACIDS

Omega-3 fatty acids like EPA and DHA have potent anti-inflammatory properties. They can reduce production of pro-inflammatory cytokines, prostaglandins, and leukotrienes.

For long COVID patients, omega-3s may mitigate lingering inflammation driving symptoms in several ways:

- They lower circulating inflammatory markers like IL-6, TNF-alpha, CRP which are often elevated for months after COVID-19 infection.

- They inhibit NF-kB activation and downstream inflammation.

- Omega-3s can dampen inflammatory signaling from the NLRP3 inflammasome implicated in long COVID.

- They reduce lipid peroxidation and oxidative stress that contributes to inflammation and symptoms.

- Omega-3s also support resolution of inflammation by enhancing maresin and resolvin synthesis. This helps prevent chronic inflammation.

The typical supplemental dosage is 1-2 grams of combined EPA/DHA daily. Omega-3s have a very favorable safety profile with minimal risk. While more research is still needed, omega-3 supplementation represents an evidence-based strategy for controlling inflammation persisting after viral illness.

Intervention	Omega-3 Fatty Acids
Suggested dose	1-2 grams EPA/DHA daily
Mechanism of action	Powerful anti-inflammatory properties, inhibits NF-kB, resolvins reduce inflammation
Evidence from other viruses	Reduced risk of developing long COVID in one study

Intervention	Omega-3 Fatty Acids
Strength of evidence	Moderate
Risk of harm	Very low

AMINO ACIDS AND HMB

Amino acids are the building blocks of proteins and play many key roles in the body. Certain amino acids may benefit long COVID patients:

- Leucine, isoleucine and valine (branched-chain amino acids) promote protein synthesis, muscle growth and energy production which may counteract long COVID muscle wasting and fatigue.

- N-acetylcysteine is a precursor to glutathione - a potent antioxidant that reduces lingering oxidative stress and supports immune function in long haulers.

- L-carnitine assists with cellular energy metabolism which may improve fatigue, brain fog and exercise intolerance.

HMB is a metabolite of the amino acid leucine. HMB:

- Stimulates muscle protein synthesis and inhibits muscle protein breakdown, helping rebuild lost muscle mass from long COVID immobilization.

- Reduces inflammation through multiple pathways including NF-kB inhibition and lowering cytokines.

- May improve mitochondrial function and energy production impaired in long haulers.

Typical dosing of HMB is 3 grams per day. Amino acids supplements should provide 2-5 grams of key ingredients like leucine, NAC, and carnitine. Amino acids and HMB supplements require further research but represent a promising approach to counteract long COVID symptoms relating to muscles, energy, and inflammation.

Intervention	Amino Acids and HMB
Suggested dose	2-5g amino acids, 3g HMB daily
Mechanism of action	Protein synthesis, anti-inflammatory, antioxidant, improve energy metabolism
Evidence from other viruses	No direct evidence
Strength of evidence	Conditional
Risk of harm	Very low

CORDYSEPS

Cordyceps is a genus of fungi used for centuries in Traditional Chinese Medicine. It contains bioactive compounds like cordycepin and polysaccharides that may benefit long COVID patients:

- Cordyceps has immunomodulating effects - regulating immune cell responses and cytokine production. This may help resolve chronic inflammation after COVID-19 infection that triggers ongoing symptoms.

- It demonstrates anti-fatigue properties in studies. In mice, cordyceps alleviates exercise-induced fatigue. This may counteract long COVID fatigue and poor endurance.

- Cordyceps improves respiratory function in research studies. It acts as a bronchodilator and lung protectant. This could benefit respiratory symptoms of long COVID.

- Antioxidant effects help reduce oxidative cellular damage from viral infections that contribute to long COVID organ impairment.

- Cordyceps may enhance mitochondrial function and energy production which is often reduced in long haulers.

Suggested dosing of cordyceps is typically 1-3 grams per day in extract form. It has a relatively positive safety profile at moderate doses. While human evidence is still limited, cordyceps represents a promising traditional supplement for managing long COVID symptoms.

Intervention	Cordyceps
Suggested dose	1-3 grams daily
Mechanism of action	Immunomodulating, anti-fatigue, antioxidant, improve respiration and energy metabolism
Evidence from other viruses	Limited evidence from in vitro and animal studies
Strength of evidence	Preliminary
Risk of harm	Low at suggested doses

COQ10/UBIQUINOL

CoQ10 is an antioxidant that supports mitochondrial function and cellular energy production. Coenzyme Q10 gets its name because it is a coenzyme - a non-protein molecule that assists enzymes in catalyzing biochemical reactions.

Specifically, CoQ10 plays a crucial role in the electron transport chain, which takes place in the inner mitochondrial membrane during cellular respiration. It participates in redox reactions that ultimately help generate ATP energy.

It may benefit long COVID patients in several ways:

- CoQ10 levels are often depleted after viral illness. Supplementation can restore optimal levels and improve fatigue, muscle weakness and brain fog common in long COVID.

- As an antioxidant, CoQ10 reduces oxidative stress that drives inflammation and symptoms in long haulers.

- It supports mitochondrial function and ATP production which is impaired in long COVID, contributing to low energy.

- CoQ10 may protect endothelial cells and lower inflammation, improving microvascular dysfunction seen in long COVID.

- It enhances cellular oxygen utilization for improved exercise performance and stamina.

The typical supplemental dosage of CoQ10 is 100-300 mg per day taken with food to enhance absorption. It is well-tolerated with minimal side effects. While more research is still needed, CoQ10 is a safe option that addresses several factors underlying long COVID based on its mechanisms.

Intervention	Coenzyme Q10
Suggested dose	100-300mg daily
Mechanism of action	Antioxidant, supports mitochondrial function, improves oxygen utilization

Intervention	Coenzyme Q10
Evidence from other viruses	No direct evidence
Strength of evidence	Conditional
Risk of harm	Very low

UBIQUINOL

- CoQ10 is the oxidized form; ubiquinol is the reduced form.

- Ubiquinol has higher bioavailability as it doesn't require conversion after ingestion.

- Ubiquinol is a stronger antioxidant than CoQ10.

- CoQ10 supplements are more common and affordable.

- CoQ10 can convert to ubiquinol in the body after absorption.

- Ubiquinol may more rapidly restore depleted CoQ10 levels.

- More research exists on CoQ10, but ubiquinol has biological advantages.

- A combination may provide optimal absorption and antioxidant effects.

In summary, ubiquinol has enhanced bioavailability and antioxidant activity, but is pricier. CoQ10 is more established but requires conversion. Overall both can increase CoQ10 levels, and a mix may give the advantages of each. More research on long COVID is still needed.

Feature	CoQ10	Ubiquinol
Form	Oxidized	Reduced
Typical dosage	100-300mg daily	50-200mg daily
Bioavailability	Lower	Higher
Antioxidant strength	Moderate	High
Cost	Low	High
Evidence for use	More established	Emerging
Long COVID rationale	Restores depleted levels, antioxidant	Enhanced absorption, potent antioxidant
Considerations	May need higher doses, convert after	Lower doses needed, limited

Feature	CoQ10	Ubiquinol
	absorbing	research

N-ACETYLCYSTEINE (NAC)

N-acetylcysteine (NAC) supports glutathione production, which has shown protective effects in animal models of influenza.

A 6-month clinical trial in 262 elderly subjects found those receiving 600 mg of NAC twice daily, versus placebo, had significantly fewer influenza-like illnesses and days spent sick in bed.

This evidence suggests supplemental NAC may provide defense against respiratory viruses like influenza. By supporting antioxidant systems, it may mitigate susceptibility and severity of illness.

However, direct evidence in COVID-19 is still lacking. More research is needed to confirm if NAC could be beneficial as an adjunctive treatment. Work closely with your healthcare provider before taking NAC supplements. Dosing, precautions, and potential drug interactions should be assessed on an individual basis.

Intervention	N-acetylcysteine (NAC)
Suggested dose	600-900 mg by mouth twice a day

Intervention	N-acetylcysteine (NAC)
Mechanism of action	Repletion of glutathione and cysteine
Evidence from other viruses	Reduced progression from colonization to illness
Strength of evidence	Limited
Risk of harm	Minimal with oral intake

ALPHA LIPOIC ACID

Alpha lipoic acid (ALA) is an antioxidant that is made by the body and found in various foods. As a supplement, it may benefit long COVID patients in the following ways:

- ALA is both fat and water soluble, allowing it to neutralize free radicals throughout cells and tissues. This helps reduce oxidative stress implicated in long COVID symptoms.

- It recycles and extends the activity of other antioxidants like vitamin C, vitamin E, and glutathione. This amplifies the antioxidant network.

- ALA modulates the NF-kB pathway to lower inflammation. This may mitigate lingering pro-inflammatory signals after COVID-19 infection.

- It enhances mitochondrial function and energy production which is often impaired in long haulers, contributing to fatigue.

- Evidence suggests ALA can protect the brain, nerves, and vascular system from oxidative damage and inflammation.

Typical ALA dosage is between 300-600 mg daily. It has a very favorable safety profile with minimal side effects at moderate doses. While human trials are still needed, ALA represents a promising antioxidant supplement to ameliorate key mechanisms underlying long COVID.

Intervention	Alpha Lipoic Acid
Suggested dose	300-600 mg daily
Mechanism of action	Powerful antioxidant, anti-inflammatory, enhances mitochondrial function
Evidence from other Viruses	No direct evidence
Strength of evidence	Theoretical basis
Risk of harm	Very low

QUERCETIN

Quercetin is a plant flavonoid that has demonstrated antiviral properties against both RNA viruses, including influenza and coronaviruses, and DNA viruses such as herpesvirus.

In addition to direct antiviral effects, quercetin also acts as a potent antioxidant and anti-inflammatory agent. It modulates signaling pathways and post-transcriptional modulators that can impact viral healing processes.

Through these pleiotropic mechanisms, quercetin may have protective effects against viral illnesses like COVID-19. Its antiviral, anti-inflammatory, and immune modulating properties could help mitigate infection severity and support recovery.

However, direct evidence in COVID-19 patients is still limited. More research is needed to confirm quercetin's clinical efficacy against SARS-CoV-2 specifically. Work closely with your healthcare provider before using quercetin supplements for COVID-19.

Intervention	Quercetin
Suggested dose	Regular: 1 gm by mouth two times a day ; Phytosome: 500 mg, two times per day
Suggested duration	Up to 12 weeks
Mechanisms of action	- Inhibits viral replication

Intervention	Quercetin
	- Modulates NLRP3 inflammasome activation
	- Modulates mast cell stabilization (anti-fibrotic)
Evidence from other viruses	Reduction of symptoms
Strength of evidence	Limited
Risk of harm	Minimal at suggested dose and duration

MELATONIN

Melatonin is a hormone produced naturally by the pineal gland that regulates sleep-wake cycles. Some research indicates it may help treat long COVID symptoms. Melatonin has strong anti-inflammatory and antioxidant properties that could reduce lingering inflammation and oxidative stress. It also helps modulate immune system activity which may be dysregulated after viral infection. Melatonin is known to improve sleep quality which could alleviate fatigue and cognitive issues associated with long COVID. Small studies show melatonin reduces headaches, anxiety, and heart palpitations in long haulers. Melatonin supplements may provide benefit, but optimal dosing is uncertain. Larger scale studies are still needed to confirm efficacy against long COVID specifically. Work closely with your healthcare provider before using melatonin.

Intervention	Melatonin
Suggested dose	5-20 mg by mouth once daily
Mechanism of action	Modulates NLRP3 inflammasome activation
Evidence from other viruses	Research in progress
Strength of evidence	Conditional
Risk of harm	Minimal

RESVERATROL

Resveratrol, a naturally occurring polyphenol, shows many beneficial health effects. It has been shown to modulate the NLRP3 inflammasome, a key mediator of inflammation. In addition, resveratrol demonstrated in vitro antiviral activity against MERS-CoV in an animal study. This suggests it may have potential to inhibit other coronaviruses like SARS-CoV-2.

Resveratrol is thought to work through multiple mechanisms. It exhibits antioxidant, anti-inflammatory, and possible antiviral properties. By modulating inflammatory pathways and inhibiting viral replication, resveratrol could mitigate viral infection severity and support recovery.

More research is still needed to determine efficacy in humans, optimal dosing, and safety. But based on early evidence, resveratrol supplementation could provide antiviral and immune-modulating benefits. Those with viral infections may want to discuss resveratrol with their healthcare provider.

Intervention	Resveratrol
Suggested Dose	100-150 mg by mouth once daily
Mechanism of Action	Modulates NLRP3 inflammasome activation
Evidence from Other Viruses	No outcomes data available
Strength of Evidence	Conditional
Risk of Harm	Minimal

Strength of Evidence	Definition
Conditional	Human trials with conflicting outcomes, or lack of published human trials. Must be supported by extensive historical experience of effectiveness, consensus of expert opinion, mechanistic plausibility, and compelling Functional Medicine model factors. In the absence of any one of these features, must be supported by compelling patient or clinical circumstances or contextual factors.
Limited	One human study demonstrating correlation between intervention and outcome, or real world data/evidence demonstrating patient oriented outcome; Must be accompanied by compelling Functional Medicine model factors and/or patient contextual factors and mechanistic plausibility.
Moderate	Two independent human studies (one of which is LOE = 1 or 2) demonstrating correlation between intervention and patient oriented outcome; mechanistic plausibility required.
Strong	Two independent human studies (both LOE = 1 or 2) demonstrating correlation between intervention and patient oriented outcome;

Strength of Evidence	Definition
	mechanistic plausibility or one additional independent human study required.

Risk of harm categories

Risk of Harm	Definition
Minimal	Risk of self-limited symptoms No risk of loss of function or corrective intervention anticipated; expected to resolve with discontinuation and observation.
Mild	Risk of self-limited symptoms. No risk of loss of function. Expected to resolve with discontinuation and minor evaluative and/or therapeutic intervention.
Significant	Risk of temporary loss of function or quality of life. Significant evaluative and/or therapeutic intervention necessary to resolve.
Severe	Risk of permanent symptoms, loss of function, quality of life, or death. Long term evaluative and/or therapeutic intervention necessary to mitigate.

About The Author

Susanna Huhtiniemi is a biochemist and functional medicine practitioner based in Southern Finland. She holds an MSc in Biochemistry from The University of Helsinki and conducted research in academic labs for several years, authoring multiple scientific publications.

Later in her career, Susanna's lifelong passion for medicine and helping others resurfaced. When her father was diagnosed with prostate cancer, she felt compelled to deepen her knowledge of how to prevent and treat chronic diseases. This motivated her to become a certified functional medicine practitioner, combining her scientific background with a functional approach to get to the root causes of illness.

In her functional medicine practice Susanna employs an investigative, root-cause approach to identify and address the underlying factors driving disease. She finds this individualized method of assessment and natural treatment to be far more effective for chronic conditions than a one-size-fits-all approach.

Susanna is fulfilled by empowering people to take charge of their own health. She believes that with the right knowledge, we can give our bodies what they need to heal and thrive. Her goal is to make this integrative approach to health and self-healing more accessible.

When she isn't working, you can find Susanna enjoying nature walks, spending time with family, and indulging her lifelong love of learning. Susanna hopes this book provides helpful new insights into improving wellbeing for readers.

ONE LAST THING...

Dear Reader,

I sincerely hope you found this book to be informative and helpful on your health journey. If you enjoyed it and feel it may benefit other readers, I would be incredibly grateful if you would consider leaving an honest review online.

Reviews empower authors like me to continue creating content that aims to educate and inspire. It also allows the book to reach more people who could use this knowledge in their own lives.

Leaving a review is easy and only takes a few minutes of your time. Simply write a few sentences about what you liked, what you learned, or how the book impacted you. And please feel free to provide constructive criticism as well - your frank feedback helps me improve.

You can leave a review on major retailer sites like Amazon where you purchased the book. You can also share your thoughts on Goodreads or social media platforms if you prefer.

Your review and support mean so much. Thank you again for giving this book a chance and for joining me on this journey to empower health. I wish you all the best!

Gratefully,
Susanna Huhtiniemi

Made in the USA
Las Vegas, NV
01 May 2024

89403645R00085